This book is needed now more than ever! Dr. Amen has written a powerful, user-friendly guide for anyone struggling with anxiety, depression, trauma, grief, or loss that will help them take control of their emotions, moods, and life. Get this book today if you want to start feeling better now.

> **MARIA MENOUNOS,** Emmy-winning journalist, *New York Times* bestselling author, and host of *Better Together with Maria Menounos* podcast

In my opinion, Dr. Daniel Amen is an undisputed leader in psychiatry by bringing forth the unique integration of neuroscience, brain imaging, and lifestyle and dietary factors as an evidence-based solution for mental illness. He has done so his entire career, and we are fortunate to have such a giant in our field. Dr. Amen's empathic brilliance shines through in all that he writes, does, and teaches. I highly recommend his new book, *Your Brain Is Always Listening*, and suggest you pick up a copy today.

> **UMA NAIDOO, MD,** director of nutritional and lifestyle psychiatry at Massachusetts General Hospital

*Your Brain Is Always Listening* blesses us with powerful, helpful strategies developed not only from Dr. Amen's decades of professional experience but also from his own recent emotional challenges. These are strategies that help us explore the deepest reaches of what underlie our moment-to-moment perceptions of the world around us and, perhaps more importantly, help us contextualize these influences and reframe how our past affects our present. This is fundamental and empowering information that we all need to embrace.

> **DAVID PERLMUTTER, MD,** author of *Brain Wash* and the #1 *New York Times* bestseller *Grain Brain*

In *Your Brain Is Always Listening*, Dr. Amen introduces a new 12-step brain-based recovery program that addresses the missing link to breaking any addiction. I highly recommend this book to anyone who has struggled with an addiction or has had trouble breaking bad habits.

> **MARK HYMAN, MD,** head of strategy and innovation, Cleveland Clinic Center for Functional Medicine; *New York Times* bestselling author of *Food Fix*

I have been a longtime fan of Dr. Amen's amazing work on the brain and recently had the honor of interviewing him on my podcast, which was a hit! He is incredibly knowledgeable, wise, and compassionate, which is exactly how I would describe his new book, *Your Brain Is Always Listening*. In a way that is both understanding and enlightening, Dr. Amen describes the many thought dragons that haunt us all and explains how changing our habits and finding true, lasting success and happiness is not only possible but achievable. I absolutely loved this book. It helped me, and I know it will help you too! I highly recommend it!

**CAROLINE LEAF, PHD,** cognitive neuroscientist and author of *Switch On Your Brain*

Dr. Amen is our most popular guest on *New Life Live!* He has helped me overcome the dragons that were attacking me and my brain. *Your Brain Is Always Listening* will help you conquer the dragons before they eat up your life.

**STEPHEN ARTERBURN,** founder of New Life Ministries and author of *Every Man's Battle*

Dr. Daniel Amen continues to support each of us with our brain health. Once again in *Your Brain Is Always Listening*, he brings us new, practical skills to support ourselves and the ones we love!

**TOM FERRY,** #1 real estate educator, bestselling author

In this book, Dr. Amen brilliantly explains why you keep doing things you don't like and exactly how to make your brain behave so it can bring you joy, peace, and fun. Read this book. Your brain is worth it!

**DAVE ASPREY,** creator of Bulletproof Coffee, three-time *New York Times* bestselling author

Dr. Amen's research into brain health and overall mental wellness is unmatched. In our rapidly changing world, it's easy to overlook how much our health, happiness, and success are controlled by the function of our brain and our associated inner dialogue. We *can* slay the dragons that limit us. But we need the right tools to do it. Everyone needs to get *Your Brain Is Always Listening* into their hands.

**SHAWN STEVENSON,** author of the international bestselling book *Sleep Smarter*

I have been associated with Dr. Amen for close to 30 years and have had the opportunity to utilize SPECT brain imaging to help so many individuals, couples, families, businesses, and ministries. *Your Brain Is Always Listening* will help you learn principles of applied neuroscience that will assist you in finding the answers you are searching for to change your brain and your life. Experienced medical and clinical psychology professionals will gain new insights into how applied neuroscience helps transform lives.

Dr. Amen has 30-plus years of brain-imaging experience that has been foundational in changing how we look at symptoms and the practical steps to take to help transform lives. Learn new insights in bringing about the desired changes in your life from a pioneer in neuroscience!

**EARL R. HENSLIN, PHD,** psychotherapist, author

# A SAMPLE OF OTHER BOOKS BY DANIEL AMEN

*The End of Mental Illness,* Tyndale, 2020

*Conquer Worry and Anxiety,* Tyndale, 2020

*Feel Better Fast and Make It Last,* Tyndale, 2018

*Memory Rescue,* Tyndale, 2017

*Stones of Remembrance,* Tyndale, 2017

*Captain Snout and the Super Power Questions,* Zonderkidz, 2017

*The Brain Warrior's Way,* with Tana Amen, New American Library, 2016

*The Brain Warrior's Way Cookbook,* with Tana Amen, New American Library, 2016

*Time for Bed, Sleepyhead,* Zonderkidz, 2016

*Change Your Brain, Change Your Life* (revised), Harmony Books, 2015, *New York Times* Bestseller

*Healing ADD* (revised), Berkley, 2013, *New York Times* Bestseller

*The Daniel Plan,* with Rick Warren, DMin, and Mark Hyman, MD, Zondervan, 2013, #1 *New York Times* Bestseller

*Unleash the Power of the Female Brain,* Harmony Books, 2013

*Use Your Brain to Change Your Age,* Crown Archetype, 2012, *New York Times* Bestseller

*Unchain Your Brain,* with David E. Smith, MD, MindWorks, 2010

*Change Your Brain, Change Your Body,* Harmony Books, 2010, *New York Times* Bestseller

*Magnificent Mind at Any Age,* Harmony Books, 2008, *New York Times* Bestseller

*The Brain in Love,* Three Rivers Press, 2007

*Making a Good Brain Great,* Harmony Books, 2005, Amazon Book of the Year

*ADD in Intimate Relationships,* MindWorks, 2005

*New Skills for Frazzled Parents,* MindWorks, 2000

# DANIEL G. AMEN, MD

# YOUR BRAIN IS ALWAYS LISTENING

## TAME THE HIDDEN DRAGONS THAT CONTROL YOUR HAPPINESS, HABITS, AND HANG-UPS

TYNDALE
MOMENTUM®

*The Tyndale nonfiction imprint*

Visit Tyndale online at tyndale.com.

Visit Tyndale Momentum online at tyndalemomentum.com.

Visit Daniel G. Amen, MD, at danielamenmd.com.

*TYNDALE*, Tyndale's quill logo, *Tyndale Momentum*, and the Tyndale Momentum logo are registered trademarks of Tyndale House Ministries. Tyndale Momentum is the nonfiction imprint of Tyndale House Publishers, Carol Stream, Illinois.

*Your Brain Is Always Listening: Tame the Hidden Dragons That Control Your Happiness, Habits, and Hang-Ups*

Designed by Mark Anthony Lane II

Published in association with the literary agency of WordServe Literary Group, www.wordserveliterary.com.

Unless otherwise indicated, all Scripture quotations are taken from the *Holy Bible*, New Living Translation, copyright © 1996, 2004, 2015 by Tyndale House Foundation. Used by permission of Tyndale House Publishers, Carol Stream, Illinois 60188. All rights reserved.

For information about special discounts for bulk purchases, please contact Tyndale House Publishers at csresponse@tyndale.com, or call 1-855-277-9400.

ISBN 978-1-4964-3820-1  (HC)
ISBN 978-1-4964-5556-7  (ITPE)

Printed in the United States of America

27   26   25   24   23   22   21
7    6    5    4    3    2

# Contents

# Introduction

## YOUR BRAIN IS ALWAYS LISTENING TO HIDDEN DRAGONS

---

*It's simply not an adventure worth telling if there aren't any dragons.*

**J. R. R. TOLKIEN**

---

In March 2020 as I was writing this book, I got a call from superstar Miley Cyrus. I could tell from the sound of her voice that she was freaking out. I'd been working with her since she was 18, when she first came to me filled with anxiety and fear. She used to worry nonstop that she would get sick or that her mom might get sick. She worried about the awful things that might happen if she didn't have a boyfriend. She even thought she would die if she wasn't in a relationship. As we worked together, Miley learned some powerful strategies to help her control these negative thoughts. But on this day, the anxiety had come roaring back, and I knew exactly why.

The coronavirus (COVID-19) outbreak, which had already killed thousands in China, was now spreading like wildfire around the globe, and it was starting to hit the US hard. On the phone, Miley rattled off so many questions about things that were terrifying her—like "How long does the virus live on packages?"—that I could hardly get a word in edgewise.

I finally managed to get Miley to take a few deep breaths with me to help her calm down. It was obvious to me that this new pandemic had unleashed Miley's dragons from the past. These long-hidden dragons were now breathing fire on the fear centers of her brain, fueling her anxiety, worry, and negative thinking patterns. I let her know that in these unprecedented times, she needed to become a dragon tamer to soothe the savage beasts within.

As we worked through the dragon taming process—the same strategies I will share with you in this book—Miley went from feeling scared and helpless to feeling empowered and in control. She couldn't wait to share what she'd learned in an Instagram Live series with her 105 million followers. She called the series *Bright Minded*, putting her own spin on my BRIGHT MINDS

1

program for better brain health, which I wrote about in *The End of Mental Illness*. I was honored to be Miley's first guest on the show, where we talked about ways to deal with the rampant stress, anxiety, depression, and loneliness, as well as the feelings of grief and loss, that were skyrocketing due to the COVID-19 pandemic.[1] From the comments her followers posted—such as "This is making me feel much better" and "Didn't know how helpful this would be. THANK YOU!"—it was clear that Miley wasn't the only one whose dragons from the past had been triggered as people were being forced to shelter at home and as the virus started crippling our economy and claiming American lives. It seemed as if everyone was feeling traumatized and mourning the loss of something—a job, a sense of security, a daily routine, a sport (playing or watching), a favorite restaurant, physical connections (no hugs!), or the death of a family member.

I had no idea at the time that COVID-19 was about to strike in my own family or that I would be suffering the devastating loss of a loved one just a few weeks later.

"She put on lipstick, wore sunglasses, packed a suitcase and, as the ambulance was arriving, she told some family members she was on her way to die." That was the opening line from an April 16, 2020, article in the *Orange County Register* about my parents and their experience with the deadly coronavirus.[2] It fit my mother perfectly. In March, my mom (Dori Amen), who was 88 at the time, and my dad (Louis Amen), who was 90, both contracted pneumonia and tested positive for COVID-19. After getting the diagnosis, medical personnel wrapped my parents in yellow tarps, loaded them into separate ambulances, and whisked them away to the hospital. I thought the future was grim. According to the Centers for Disease Control (CDC), 10 to 27 percent of seniors over the age of 85 who develop the illness will die.[3] I was afraid my parents might be among them.

My parents' doctor, also the hospital's infectious disease director, admitted in the *Register* article that when my parents arrived at the hospital, he was petrified. But he had not met my mom and dad. Five days later, my parents left the hospital COVID-free and went home. It appeared they had beaten the illness. Over the next few weeks, my mom recovered quickly and really wanted to get back to playing golf, but my father continued to struggle. He had been suffering from a cough for weeks prior to testing positive for COVID-19, and he had recently been in the hospital for a gastrointestinal bleed that caused him to lose one-quarter of his blood.

On May 5, 2020, as I was getting ready to pick him up for a follow-up appointment, my mom called me in a panic saying he wasn't breathing. I dialed 911 and raced over to their home. The paramedics did their best, but they couldn't get him breathing again.

My dad joined the angels that day.

And suddenly the Grief and Loss Dragons that I had been helping so many of my patients and social media followers cope with during the pandemic unleashed a fireball in my brain. Fortunately, as a psychiatrist who has spent decades helping people deal with death and loss, I knew that I needed to start the healing process as soon as possible. Some people think you need to wallow in suffering following the death of a loved one, but I always ask, "If you broke your arm, would you wait six weeks to get the bone set?" One of the most important steps in healthy grieving—I'll go over all of the steps in more detail in section 1 on the Death Dragons and the Grief and Loss Dragons—is to express your feelings rather than bottling them up. So I decided to share my pain with my followers on social media.

In a series of nightly live chats during the pandemic, I explained that during the mourning process—and at all times—your brain is always listening and responding to the hidden influences that act on it. This became even more evident in May 2020 when the heartbreaking and senseless death of George Floyd—a black man from Minneapolis who was killed when a white police officer kneeled on his neck for over eight minutes despite his cries of "I can't breathe"—led to rage and destruction. This social injustice on top of the rampant stress of the pandemic triggered the release of Angry, Judgmental, and Ancestral Dragons (which you will learn more about in this book) that drove some people into the streets to protest peacefully while spurring others to loot, vandalize, and set fires. The powerful influences on your brain include:

- *Dragons from the Past*—memories and events that still breathe fire on your emotional centers, driving your behavior

- *They, Them, and Other Dragons*—other people in your life—past and present—who each have their own set of dragons

- *ANTs*—automatic negative thoughts that link, stack, and attack you, providing the fuel for anxiety and depression

- *Bad Habit Dragons*—habits that result from dragon influences and increase the chances you'll be overweight and depressed, and have brain fog

- *Scheming Dragons*—advertisers, news feeds, social media sites, and the gadgets in your pocket that steal your mind and money

- *Addicted Dragons*—repetitive behaviors that damage your health, wealth, or relationships

Unless you recognize and redirect these influences, they can steal your happiness, damage your relationships, pilfer your health, rob your ability to cope with stress (like the coronavirus pandemic), and limit your destiny. The good news is that once you become aware and tame these dragons and eliminate the ANTs, you can break bad habits, shut down self-defeating thoughts, shore up your capacity to cope with uncertainty, reduce your vulnerability to schemers, and heal addictions. In fact, taming your dragons is essential for good mental health because when they control your brain, your entire life suffers.

## JIMMY'S HIDDEN DRAGONS

The afternoon I met Jimmy, 39, a high-level business executive, he sat next to his wife on the soft burgundy leather sofa in my office. He had just been released from a psychiatric hospital that morning and looked anxious and worn-out. A week prior he'd told an emergency room doctor he had thought of killing himself to end the feelings of dread, panic, anxiety, and hopelessness that just wouldn't go away. His Anxious Dragon, one of the 13 Dragons from the Past, was running rampant in his brain.

Jimmy had been seeing another psychiatrist for years to refill medication for anxiety and depression, which was explained as "working to fix a chemical imbalance." The medication took the edge off his negative feelings, but it also took the edge off his positive feelings. While seeing the psychiatrist, he never learned any skills to deal with his Anxious Dragons or the 12 other ones that fueled his dark thoughts and mood swings.

The current "episode" that brought Jimmy to the ER started two weeks before when he found out he had to give a presentation to one of his company's largest customers. It filled him with dread. He told me, "If I had to describe the fear, it's like you're on death row and the clock's run out. The guard opens the door and you must take the first step—that kind of fear runs through my bones." Jimmy had struggled with glossophobia (the fear of public speaking) since middle school. Through an exercise called Break the Bonds of the Past, which I will explain later, we learned that this fear started when he was 12, the day his grandmother made him give an "impact statement" at the Los Angeles County Superior Court about why his father, one of the leaders of a violent street gang, should not get the death penalty for a double homicide. Jimmy's Anxious Dragons breathed fire on the fear centers in his young brain, and he was attacked by ANTs (automatic negative thoughts), including, *What if I cannot speak in court and end up killing my father?*

Even though Jimmy had repressed the memory, his Anxious Dragons haunted him throughout the rest of middle school, high school, and college, and into his adult life. He went to great lengths to avoid waking these dragons by dodging any presentations until about six years before when his supervisor asked him to give a brief talk at work about his role in the company. He loved his job but ruminated for days about how he would be unable to put his thoughts into words. Even after giving the presentation, the ANTs multiplied, stacked on top of one another, and attacked him, linking to many other catastrophic thoughts, such as:

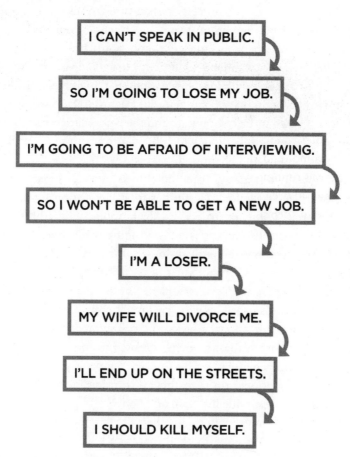

That is when Jimmy started to see his original psychiatrist, went on medication, and made a conscious decision to overcome his fear, which worked for a while. He gave tours at work, traveled, and met with clients. He also gave his life to God and became an active member of his church, which he found incredibly helpful. However, the Anxious Dragons and other Dragons from the Past reappeared when he was given new responsibility at work, and once again his anxiety spiraled out of control.

Growing up, Jimmy had experienced intense, persistent psychological trauma (Wounded Dragons). He saw his father dealing drugs and beating up people. His father was incarcerated when Jimmy was a small child, and he went with his grandmother to visit his dad, who made him introduce himself to other gang leaders, which filled Jimmy with dread. He witnessed drive-by shootings and was in car chases before age nine. He was kidnapped twice by feuding family members, and he feared for his life on many occasions. Once a dozen SWAT officers crashed through his family's front door with weapons drawn while Jimmy was lying on the couch in his father's arms during a rare time when his father was home on parole. After his father's rearrest, his mother sent Jimmy to live with his grandparents, even though she kept his two younger siblings. His Abandoned, Invisible, or Insignificant Dragons told his brain that he was alone and unloved. He also witnessed his grandmother being sexually assaulted, and the perpetrator asked Jimmy if he wanted to have sex with her too, which filled him with a sense of shame and hopelessness (Should and Shaming Dragons).

Jimmy's brain was always listening to his Ancestral Dragons from his family history and genetics. His mother took medication for anxiety, and there was a family history of anxiety and alcohol abuse. His father's side of the family had rampant psychiatric issues, including panic attacks, depression, and drug abuse, and his siblings had similar problems.

Jimmy's brain was also always listening to his Bad Habit Dragons that had formed from listening to the other dragons in his life. One of Jimmy's bad habits particularly disturbed his wife. He loved to watch violent movies, boxing and UFC matches, animal attacks, and execution documentaries, which he had watched with his father. Being exposed to intense, life-threatening violence as a young child had set his "arousal template" (what gave him the most powerful emotional rush) to these disturbing images, but they only perpetuated the stress inside his brain and body.

Not only was Jimmy's brain run by these dragons, he'd also had a number of head injuries from playing football (he was a high school all-conference linebacker), boxing until he was 18, and being involved in a number of bar fights. When he was 15, he fell eight feet onto his head; he convulsed, lost consciousness for about 10 minutes, and lost the hearing in his right ear. He was hospitalized for four days, and that whole summer he had to relearn how to walk. To quiet his Anxious and Wounded Dragons, Jimmy used drugs and alcohol as a teenager and young adult, but they gave him only temporary relief.

Jimmy had no idea that dragons were running his brain and his life. The only messages his brain could hear were that he was hopeless, messed up, and a failure. Jimmy's dragons told him many stories—such as *You were abandoned*, *You are unlovable*, *The world is dangerous*, and *You can't speak in public*—which eventually caused his downward spiral and his belief that he'd be better off dead. Most of us did not have trauma as intense as Jimmy's growing up, but unless we are consciously taught how to identify the voices of our dragons, we may still create horror stories based on erroneous or incomplete inputs that can cause us to feel or act in self-defeating ways.

As part of our evaluation of Jimmy, we took a detailed history to understand the story of his life, reviewed the records from his prior doctor and the hospital, ran a complete set of laboratory tests, and did a sophisticated 3D brain imaging study called SPECT (single photon emission computed tomography), which is a nuclear medicine study that evaluates brain blood flow and activity. SPECT is different from the structural CT or MRI scans, which both assess brain anatomy. SPECT looks at how the brain functions and basically tells us three things about brain activity: whether it is healthy, underactive, or overactive. At Amen Clinics we have been performing SPECT scans for 30 years and have built the world's largest database of brain scans related to mental health issues, totaling more than 175,000 scans on patients from 155 countries.

The images on the following page represent a healthy SPECT scan. The image on the left looks at the outside surface of the brain, which shows full, even, symmetrical activity. It's called a surface scan. In the image on the right, white shows the most active areas. In a healthy scan these are typically in the cerebellum (the back, bottom part of the brain), which contains half the brain's neurons. The image on the right is called an active scan.

## REPRESENTATIVE HEALTHY SPECT SCANS

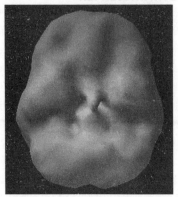 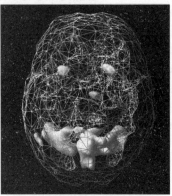

Underside surface scan
Full, even, symmetrical activity

Underside active scan
White equals most active parts
of the brain, typically in the
cerebellum in back, bottom area

## JIMMY'S SPECT SCANS

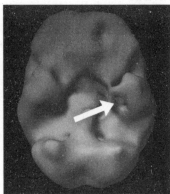 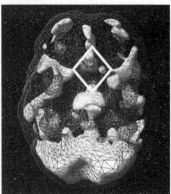

Underside surface scan
Damage to left temporal lobe

Active scan
Diamond pattern of activation in
emotional areas of brain

Jimmy's SPECT scan showed two significant findings:

1. Low activity in his left temporal lobe on the surface scan, in a pattern consistent with past brain trauma. This part of the brain is involved with mood stability, irritability, expressive language difficulties (finding the right words), memory issues, anxiety, and dark thoughts. When hurt, this area can send interruption signals to the rest of the brain.

2. Increased activity in a diamond pattern in the limbic or emotional part of the brain, consistent with past emotional trauma that became stuck in his brain, so it is always listening to painful inputs from the past.

By diligently using the strategies in this book, by understanding and taming the hidden dragons and eliminating the ANTs, and by getting his diet, nutrients, and brain healthy, Jimmy thrived. Over the next six months, his mood stabilized and his anxiety lessened. He was able to become an even more important part of his team at work and a happier and more loving husband and father. In addition, he lost 37 pounds, felt stronger, and had more energy than he'd had in years. He also started to help others in his family get well. Continuing to use these strategies during the pandemic helped him and his family cope in healthy ways that kept them emotionally strong in spite of the added stress.

This book will explore the many reasons—some hidden and some obvious (like the pandemic)—that dragons and ANTs are constantly talking to your brain, making you feel sad, anxious, worried, depressed, mad, or out of control. With practical strategies to tame your dragons, you will take control of your brain and be able to choose what it listens to. You'll no longer give in to negative thinking or let bad habits derail your health and relationships even in times of trauma, extreme stress, or grief. You'll be able to recognize what's true, build your self-confidence, discipline your mind, and feel happier, calmer, and in more control of your own destiny. In order to get and stay well, once you understand and use this information, share it with loved ones; that way you are also creating your own support group, making it more likely you will keep these new habits for the rest of your life.

# Your Brain

*A Very Brief Primer*

As we embark on this journey together, it's important to briefly get acquainted with six brain systems involved in running your life. I will refer to them many times throughout this book, and I want you to have a quick reference for them here. Obviously, your brain is complicated and involves many structures, but these are particularly important as they work in concert to create your moods, anxieties, memory, and behavior.

## INSIDE VIEW OF THE BRAIN

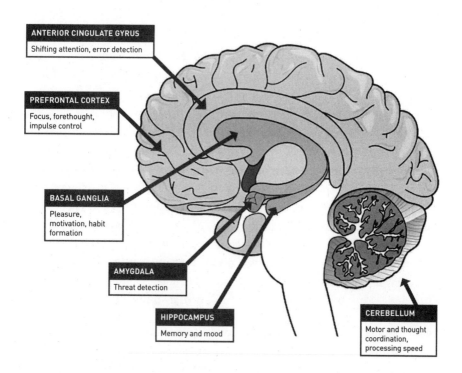

**ANTERIOR CINGULATE GYRUS**
Shifting attention, error detection

**PREFRONTAL CORTEX**
Focus, forethought, impulse control

**BASAL GANGLIA**
Pleasure, motivation, habit formation

**AMYGDALA**
Threat detection

**HIPPOCAMPUS**
Memory and mood

**CEREBELLUM**
Motor and thought coordination, processing speed

**Prefrontal cortex (PFC):** Found in the front third of the brain, the PFC plays a major role in executive functions (like the boss at work), such as focus, forethought, judgment, planning, decision making, and impulse control. When it is low in activity from head trauma, toxins, attention deficit hyperactivity disorder (ADHD), or other causes, people tend to struggle with attention, distractibility, disorganization, procrastination, and impulsive behavior. It is like the boss went on vacation.

**Anterior cingulate gyrus (ACG):** Found deep within the frontal lobes, it is involved with shifting attention and error detection. When the ACG is overactive, people tend to struggle with getting stuck on negative thoughts or behaviors, worrying, being oppositional or argumentative, or seeing too many errors in themselves or others.

**Amygdala (AMY):** This almond-shaped structure is found underneath the temples and behind the eyes; there is one on each side of the brain. They are involved in emotion, threat detection, and aggression. They tend to be overactive in people who have past emotional trauma, are hypervigilant (always watching for something bad to happen), and are socially anxious. When the AMY are underactive, people tend to have less fear, like the rock climber in *Free Solo*, and be risk-takers.

**Hippocampus (HC):** Greek for "seahorse" (*hippo*—horse; *kampos*—sea monster), your two hippocampi are about the size of your thumbs and found deep in the brain on the inside of your left and right temporal lobes, just behind the amygdala. They are part of your emotional brain and help you feel happy or sad and are central to memory. They retain new information and store it for up to several weeks; if it is reinforced, you keep it longer. If the hippocampi (plural) are damaged, you cannot store new information. In the movie *50 First Dates*, Lucy, Drew Barrymore's character, had a severe car accident that damaged her left and right hippocampi. After she falls asleep, memories of the prior day are wiped out. Memory problems are associated with low activity in the HC, and it is one of the first areas of the brain that dies in Alzheimer's disease. The HC also can produce up to 700 new stem cells a day if put in a nourishing environment (think good nutrition, omega-3 fatty acids, oxygen levels, blood flow, and mental stimulation).[1]

**Basal ganglia (BG):** These large structures deep in the brain are involved in habit formation. The BG also contain the nucleus accumbens (NA), which is part of your reward system (motivates you to go toward pleasure and away from pain), and is exquisitely responsive to the feel-good neurotransmitter dopamine, involved in addictions. The NA is involved with cravings, and if it is underactive, people tend to feel flat and depressed, and they are more vulnerable to addiction and craving substances that activate it, such as drugs, alcohol, sex, or high-calorie sugary foods.

**Cerebellum (CB):** Latin for "little brain," it is located at the back, bottom portion of the brain. It is only 10 percent of the brain's volume, yet it contains half of the brain's neurons or cells. It is involved in coordination, processing speed, language, cognitive processing, and language.

## THE FOUR CIRCLES OF HEALTH AND ILLNESS

These biological systems of the brain represent one of four circles of overall physical and mental health, which I think about whenever I evaluate or treat any patient. I first wrote about them in my book *Change Your Brain, Change Your Life.*[2]

**B** **Biological:** how the physical aspects of your brain and body function. One of the major principles of my work is that if you want to keep the physical functioning of your brain healthy or rescue it if it is headed for trouble, you have to prevent or treat the 11 major risk factors that steal your mind. My team created the mnemonic BRIGHT MINDS to summarize them: blood flow, retirement/aging, inflammation, genetics, head trauma, toxins, mind storms (abnormal electrical activity), immunity and infections (relevant for a pandemic), neurohormones, diabesity (a combination of being overweight and having high blood sugar), and sleep disturbances.[3] The biological circle also encompasses diet and exercise.

**P** **Psychological:** how you think and talk to yourself, as well as self-concept, body image, emotional trauma, upbringing, and significant life events (such as enduring months of self-isolation during the coronavirus pandemic). Dragons influence your psychological health by saying whether you are enough—good enough, smart enough, pretty enough, strong enough, rich enough, and so on. When you've tamed your dragons and believe that you are enough, you will be happier and more confident. When you feel less than enough, your brain can give in to sadness, anxiety, and failure.

**S** Social: the quality of your relationships and any current life stresses. When you have solid relationships, a healthy family, a role or career you enjoy, and financial stability, your brain tends to do much better than when any of these areas are troubled. Dragons can become unhinged when difficult life situations, such as a global pandemic, relationship breakup or divorce, layoff, or death of a loved one, elevate stress hormone levels. When this circle is unhealthy, you are more vulnerable to illnesses, including infections like COVID-19, as well as depression, anxiety disorders, and more.

**SP** Spiritual: your connection to God, the planet, and past and future generations; and your deepest sense of meaning and purpose. You are more than just your brain cells, thoughts, and connections. I believe we are all created with divine purpose. When your brain listens to dragons or ANTs, it's easy to forget that your life matters and you have a role and a calling to fulfill.

When any one circle is unhealthy, your brain is more likely to listen to your Dragons from the Past, from others, and from society, and then let them take control.

Jimmy's biological circle included prior head traumas, genetic vulnerability inherited from his parents, toxins from past substance abuse, mind storms (abnormal temporal lobes), and diabesity (high blood sugar plus excess weight). His psychological circle was loaded with Dragons from the Past, ANTs, and developmental trauma. His social circle struggled with abandonment issues and work-related stress (expectation to speak in public). His spiritual circle was a source of strength that helped ameliorate his pain. With steps to improve his health in the four circles, we were able to heal his brain, tame his dragons, and help his brain start listening to healthier messages. I'll help you do the same.

# TAME THE DRAGONS FROM THE PAST

## YOUR HISTORY IS NOT YOUR DESTINY

---

*People who deny the existence of dragons are often eaten by dragons from within.*

URSULA K. LE GUIN, *THE WAVE IN THE MIND*

---

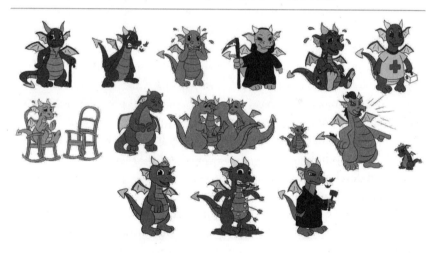

Since the beginning of time, we have communicated with each other through stories. They help us understand our place in the world and teach us how to act or not act. They shape our perceptions and pass down knowledge and morals. Personal stories guide and direct our lives. How we interpret our experiences is one of the driving forces behind happiness or depression, exhilaration or disappointment, rage or peace. Telling our personal stories is something we do every day by how we think, feel, behave, and interact with others. Every conversation we have is, in some way or another, a reflection of the stories we've created over time. These stories create the movies that are constantly playing in our heads—"I am a good mother . . . a bad father . . . an alcoholic . . . a success . . . a victim . . . a fool."

## THE *DRAGONS FROM THE PAST*

My friend Dr. Sharon May, a world-renowned relationship psychologist, calls the stories that interfere with our lives Dragons from the Past that are still breathing fire on our amygdala (the almond-shaped structure on the inside of your temporal lobes involved in emotional reactions), driving anxiety, anger, irrational behavior, and automatic negative reactions. On an episode of *The Brain Warrior's Way Podcast* that I cohost with my wife, Tana, Dr. May said, "All of us have Dragons from the Past influencing our present feelings and actions."[1] Unless you recognize and tame them, and consciously calm and protect your amygdala from overfiring, these dragons will haunt your unconscious mind and drive emotional pain for the rest of your life. What blows from an ember, or a small action of another, can turn into a destructive fire of anxiety and rage.

After learning from Dr. May, I started using this concept with my patients, including Jimmy. Over time I identified 13 Dragons from the Past, including their origins, triggers that make them overpowering, and how they cause us to react. All of us have more than one Dragon from the Past driving our behavior, and they are always interacting with the Dragons from the Past of others, causing both internal and external battles—a modern-day *Game of Thrones*. All of us have primary and secondary dragons driving our behavior. Primary ones are present most of the time, while secondary ones come out during times of stress, such as the COVID-19 pandemic that began in 2020. You'll learn which ones apply to you. (You can also take the Hidden Dragons quiz at KnowYourDragons.com.)

# DRAGONS FROM THE PAST

1. Abandoned, Invisible, or Insignificant Dragons—feel alone, unseen, or unimportant
2. Inferior or Flawed Dragons—feel inferior to others
3. Anxious Dragons—feel fearful and overwhelmed
4. Wounded Dragons—bruised by past trauma
5. Should and Shaming Dragons—racked with guilt
6. Special, Spoiled, or Entitled Dragons—feel more special than others
7. Responsible Dragons—need to take care of others
8. Angry Dragons—harbor hurts and rage
9. Judgmental Dragons—hold harsh or critical opinions of others due to past injustices
10. Death Dragons—fear the future and lack of a meaningful life
11. Grief and Loss Dragons—feel loss and fear of loss
12. Hopeless and Helpless Dragons—have pervasive sense of despair and discouragement
13. Ancestral Dragons—affected by issues from past generations

I will show you how to tame your dragons with four specific strategies and rewrite the stories they've been telling you. You'll learn to recognize where they came from, what triggers them, and how they react. I'll show you upsides if there are any, and I'll give you a group of affirmations to say or meditate on each day to soothe and calm the dragons. I'll share some of my own Dragons from the Past and how they've tortured me, influenced me, and fueled some of my success. Self-disclosure has been a useful tool in helping my patients so they know that I see myself as a fellow traveler and guide in the "mind" fields of our lives. Plus, as a fun exercise, I imagine the type of movies each dragon species might like and give some examples.

# ABANDONED, INVISIBLE, OR INSIGNIFICANT DRAGONS

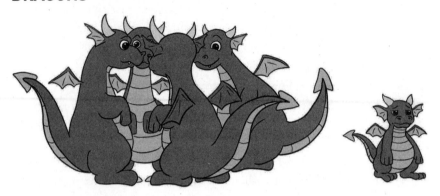

**Origin:** Others did not see or recognize you, or you felt unimportant, abandoned, and lonely. These dragons are common in children whose parents were unable or unavailable to raise them. They are also common in middle children from large families and those whose parents or siblings were dysfunctional, narcissistic (all about them), or sick. These dragons also occur in families where one of the parents or siblings was a high achiever or famous. The other spouse or children often felt invisible or unloved by comparison.

**Triggers:** When you perceive that others ignore or belittle you; when others are recognized and you are not; when you get laid off from work but your colleagues don't.

**Reactions:** These dragons fire up loneliness, worthlessness, or feeling small. They can also lead to an inflated sense of importance to make up for feeling insignificant. They are associated with abandonment issues and cause people to commit to relationships too quickly before taking time to assess the health of a relationship. They can also cause jealousy and unwarranted insecurities and pain. Many relationship issues happen when your Abandoned, Invisible, or Insignificant Dragons breathe fire on your emotional brain regions, causing you to overreact. If you are dealing with another person who has these same dragons, it can cause a war that destroys the relationship.

**Movies:** These dragons love underdog movies, such as *Rocky, Rudy, Gladiator, 300, The Karate Kid, The Blind Side*, or *Slumdog Millionaire*.

**Daniel's Abandoned, Invisible, or Insignificant Dragons:** This is my primary dragon. I'm the third of seven children, with an older sister and brother, and four younger sisters. My wife, Tana, grew up with a lot of drama and trauma, and by her estimation, my home was akin to the television shows of the fifties and sixties: *Donna Reed, Father Knows Best,* and *Leave It to Beaver.* Yet many of the stories or dragons I developed for myself as a child were distressing and unhelpful.

Being a middle child and the second son in a Lebanese family meant I often felt insignificant. My father owned a chain of grocery stores, and in Middle Eastern families, the oldest son is expected to go into the family business. That meant my brother was "the chosen one," and I was not.

With so many children, our parents had little time for individual attention. My father worked 80 or more hours a week, driven by his Anxious Dragons that were born during the Great Depression. I didn't see much of him until I was 10 years old and could go to work with him on weekends. But at work, he wasn't my dad; he was my boss. My mother was always busy cooking, cleaning, and getting us from place to place. I coveted the 20 minutes a week I read with her, but I often felt invisible.

My Abandoned, Invisible, or Insignificant Dragons drove me to want to be connected, seen, and significant. I've worked hard over the course of my life to make a difference in others, and I love sharing what I have learned in front of large crowds. One of my favorite lectures ever was at the American Airlines Arena in front of 20,000 people. In large part, these dragons are why I am writing this book.

### *Tools to tame your Abandoned, Invisible, or Insignificant Dragons*

1. **Do you recognize Abandoned, Invisible, or Insignificant Dragons in your life?** Do you feel overlooked, unimportant, or lonely? Did you grow up in a large family? Did your parents divorce when you were young, were they absent or neglectful, were you adopted, or did you bounce around in foster care?

2. **Find the upside:** These dragons may drive you to be significant and help others, to become part of a group that brings positive energy to the world. The upside of these dragons for me was freedom. Since I was not the oldest male child in my Lebanese family, I had the choice to do anything I wanted with my life. I didn't love the grocery business, but I have loved being a psychiatrist and author for the last 40 years. Rather than being jealous of my older brother, I have immense gratitude for him.

3. **Strategies:**

**Know your life's purpose.** You will feel more significant, happy, and connected. Business executive Adam Leipzig gives one of my favorite online talks about finding your purpose in just five minutes.[2] He starts by telling a story about his 25th college reunion from Yale University where he made an astounding discovery: 80 percent of his privileged, well-off, powerful friends were unhappy with their lives, despite being on their second spouses and second houses. The difference between them and those who were happy was "knowing their purpose." To know your purpose, he says, you have to know the answers to five simple questions:

1. Who are you? What is your name?

2. What do you love to do? Examples include writing, cooking, designing, creating, speaking, teaching, crunching numbers, etc. To get clarity of purpose, ask yourself, *What is the one thing I do that I feel qualified to teach others?*

3. Whom do you do it for? Or how does your work connect you to others?

4. What do those people want or need from you?

5. How do they change as a result of what you do?

When I answer these questions, it looks like this:

1. My name is Daniel.

2. I love optimizing people's brains and inspiring them to care about brain health.

3. I do it for my family and for those who come to our clinics, read my books, follow our social media channels, or watch our public television shows.

4. The people I touch want to suffer less, feel better, be sharper, and have greater control over their lives. They want better brains and better lives.

5. As a result of what I do, people change by having better brains and better lives; they suffer less and become happier, and they pass on what they've learned about brain health to others.

Notice that only two of the five questions are about you; three are about others. A wise Chinese saying is: "If you want happiness for an hour, take a nap. If you want happiness for a day, go fishing. If you want happiness for a year, inherit a fortune. If you want happiness for a lifetime, help somebody." Happiness is found in helping others.

When you're at a gathering and someone asks you, "What do you do?" give them the answer to question number five. In my example, when people ask me what I do, I say, "I help people have better brains and better lives, so they suffer less, become happier, and pass it on to others." By answering that simple question, I get to share my life purpose and quiet my Abandoned, Invisible, or Insignificant Dragons. What is your purpose?

**Work toward making a difference in the lives of others.** Volunteering actually helps to grow the hippocampus (memory and mood) and improves a person's sense of achievement and productivity over a two-year period.[3]

**Become part of a group (church, civic, environmental, etc.).** Being socially connected is critical to staying healthy. Humans are not polar bears; we are a species that needs one another. Find creative ways to connect if you can't meet in person. At the start of the pandemic, government officials began talking about the need for social distancing. I knew immediately it was a bad term. The term should have been physical distancing, which is what is needed to stop spreading the virus. In such a crisis, we need to be socially connected more than ever before, and the accurate use of language matters, as we will see in the chapter on taming our thoughts.

**Psychotherapy can be very helpful**, especially for abandonment issues. Be careful not to run away from therapy too soon. When you get close to the therapist, it may make you nervous and want to run, which may also be a pattern in relationships.

4. **Affirmations to say or meditate on every day:**

I am loved.
I am unique.
I am significant.
I am seen by . . . [name the people who see you].
I am making a difference in the lives of . . . [name them].

## INFERIOR OR FLAWED DRAGONS

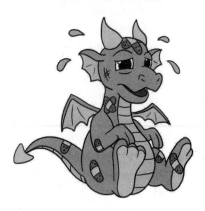

**Origin:** You felt "less than" others in ability, looks, money, achievement, or relationships. You felt inadequate or that you could not live up to your parents' expectations. You were bullied, cut down, or criticized by peers, family, or authority figures, or you frequently compared yourself to others in a negative way. *Due to social media, these dragons are causing an epidemic rise of anxiety, depression, and suicide in young people.*

**Triggers:** When you compare yourself to others or compete against others; when you look in the mirror.

**Reactions:** These dragons drive feelings of inferiority, depression, helplessness, and jealousy; make you overly sensitive or a perfectionist; may lead to impostor syndrome (feeling like a fraud or you don't know what you're doing) or body dysmorphic disorder, where you see only your body's flaws.

**Movies:** These dragons love superhero movies, especially ones with Marvel X-Men mutant characters who have special powers.

**Daniel's Inferior or Flawed Dragons:** This is a secondary dragon for me. I was short and thought I was funny looking: My mom is five feet tall, and my father was about five feet six inches, which is where I ended up. I was usually the smallest kid in the class, and because of this, I was teased, was picked last for sports activities, and felt "less than" other boys. Given all the girls in my family, my mother did not have time to comb the boys' hair every morning, so my brother and I had butch haircuts during elementary school. Mix that with the big ears I inherited from my grandfather, and I was often called Dumbo.

Early on, I never felt smart. I went to a Catholic elementary school that had 48 children in each class (six rows across, eight desks deep) and never stood out academically. My parents were so busy that my school performance was not a priority as long as I wasn't failing.

Not being able to live up to successful parents or older siblings often makes people feel inadequate. My father was the embodiment of the American dream. Coming from poor immigrant parents, he rose to build a 100-million-dollar grocery chain business. When I was young, I knew he was a successful businessman. Successful parents are not always a blessing because children often compare themselves to their parents or siblings and wonder if they can measure up. Self-esteem is the difference between where you believe you are and where you think you should be compared to others. If they match, you tend to feel good about yourself. If they don't match, you feel inferior.

---

*Self-esteem is the difference between where you believe you are and where you think you should be.*

---

These dragons fueled much of my success. Over time I realized that being shorter meant every seat on an airplane has first-class legroom, I never hit my head on doorjambs, and people are drawn to me ultimately because of who I am as a person, not my size. I would have rather been six feet eight inches so I could have played for the Los Angeles Lakers, but because of my brain, I was able to spend a year with the NBA, training their referees about brain health. Plus, I was the primary investigator in the world's first and largest brain imaging and rehabilitation study on active and retired NFL players. They towered over me, but I was able to help many have better brains and better lives. Plus, with the brain damage I saw on their scans, I am more grateful than ever that I was only a backup quarterback in high school, which turned out to be the safest position on the field.

Since I was not exceptionally smart, I learned to work hard. I still consider my late father to be one of the most successful people I have ever known, but through consistent effort over time, I've been able to leave my own mark for my family and the people we serve.

---

*Comparison is the thief of joy.*

**THEODORE ROOSEVELT**

---

*Tools to tame your Inferior or Flawed Dragons*

1. **Do you recognize Inferior or Flawed Dragons in your life?** Do you have a tendency to compare yourself to others or find yourself envious? Do you feel less than others? Do you feel like you are not enough? Have you faced a lot of verbal put-downs from others?

2. **Find the upside:** If you were perfect, you'd be God—and, clearly, you're not. Accepting your flaws will help you accept others because we all have flaws. This can help you be more humble and compassionate.

3. **Strategies:** Arianna Huffington calls these dragons "the obnoxious roommate in your head" and says to "give them an eviction notice!"[4]

   **Work hard to stop comparing yourself to others, and be the best you can be.** You can do this by:

   1. Being aware when you do it

   2. Knowing what triggers you to compare yourself to others and avoiding them (e.g., social media, magazine/TV ads)

   3. Changing your focus to something else

   4. Focusing on your strengths and accomplishments

   5. Praising others because it makes it more likely you will praise yourself

   6. Avoiding mindlessly scrolling through social media. On one of our *Brain Warrior's Way Podcast* episodes, my cohost and wife, Tana, relayed the story of doing Christmas shopping online, where she saw an image of another woman her age who looked perfect. She immediately started to feel inferior and thought of searching for plastic surgery sites. Thankfully, she recognized the dragons whispering to her brain and pulled herself away.

   **Stop caring what other people think of you because they are mostly *not* thinking about you at all.** I teach my patients the 18-40-60 rule: When you're 18, you worry about what everyone else is thinking of you; when you're 40, you don't care what anyone else is thinking about you; and when you're 60, you realize no one has been thinking about you at all. People spend their days worrying and thinking about themselves, not you.

**Realize that seeking perfection is a reason to fail** and that when you constantly compare yourself to others, you are doomed to unhappiness. There will always be someone healthier, richer, prettier, bigger, or stronger than you. There will also always be someone poorer, uglier, smaller, and weaker than you. Where you bring your attention determines how you feel. Comparing yourself negatively to others, which society and social media promote, is a trap that damages many people. Don't be one of them.

4. **Affirmations to say or meditate on every day:**

I am unique.
I restrain comparing myself to others.
I am a strong, independent person.
I will be my best, not someone else's best.
I work hard.

## ANXIOUS DRAGONS

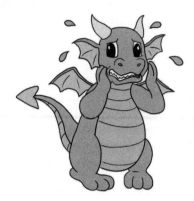

**Origin:** You were often afraid, had a sense of impending doom, felt overwhelmed or stressed, or thought the world was a dangerous place, causing you to develop anxiety and/or security issues. Having an alcoholic, drug-addicted, angry, or unpredictable parent, stepparent, or sibling can create these dragons. These are the most common Dragons from the Past, as 31 percent of the US population will experience an anxiety disorder at some point in life.[5] Living through the coronavirus pandemic has certainly spawned millions more of these dragons around the world. According to a report published in April 2020, the number of prescriptions filled for anti-anxiety medications spiked more than 34 percent in just one month early that year.[6]

**Triggers:** When you are reminded in any way of situations from the past that caused anxiety, like the palpable fear and uncertainty of a global pandemic, or more everyday occurrences, such as a negative look from someone important to you, having to speak in public, hearing a loud noise, or being overscheduled.

**Reactions:** These dragons drive panic attacks (intense, unexpected fear) and nervousness; predict the worst; and cause physical stress symptoms, phobias, and worry about safety issues or being scrutinized. These dragons lead you to avoid conflict, public places, and known stressful situations. If this is your primary dragon, you may lack confidence in your abilities; be shy, timid, or easily embarrassed; or be sensitive to criticism. These dragons may also lead to self-destructive behaviors, such as drug or alcohol abuse, to escape the anxious feelings. Here are other common symptoms of the Anxious Dragons:

Heightened muscle tension (headaches, sore muscles, hand tremors)
Periods of heart pounding, rapid heart rate, or chest pain

Periods of trouble breathing or feeling smothered
Periods of feeling dizzy, faint, or unsteady on your feet
Periods of nausea or abdominal upset
Periods of sweating, or hot or cold flashes
Tics (motor or vocal)
Tendency to freeze in anxiety-provoking situations
Fingernail biting or skin picking

**Movies:** These dragons hate horror movies but tend to love funny, uplifting movies like *Mrs. Doubtfire*, *Big*, *Chef*, and Disney's *Pollyanna*.

**Daniel's Anxious Dragons:** I wet my bed at night until I was about nine years old. Every morning, I woke up in a panic, not knowing if the sheets would be wet, which caused my brain to become hypervigilant and always be on guard looking for trouble. I also bit my fingernails, often until they bled, a bad habit that took me many years to break.

Growing up in the fifties and sixties was not all *Donna Reed* and *Leave It to Beaver*. As a child, I remember many "air-raid drills," where we had to take shelter under our desks, preparing for nuclear bombs from the Soviet Union. We also had earthquake drills, which were practical since we lived near the epicenter of the 1971 San Fernando earthquake. Plus, the Vietnam War was raging from the time I was ten, and I recall older siblings of my friends dying. I had a low draft number and became an infantry medic myself. I never got used to being shot at.

The anxiety stemming from my youth was one reason I fell in love with teaching my patients relaxation techniques, such as diaphragmatic breathing, guided imagery, and hypnosis. They helped reset my nervous system, which made me more effective at helping our patients. They also helped me better cope with the uncertainty and fear of the coronavirus pandemic.

*Tools to tame your Anxious Dragons*

1. **Do you recognize Anxious Dragons in your life?** Do you have any of the common emotional reactions or physical symptoms of Anxious Dragons?

2. **Find the upside:** Anxious Dragons can lead people to develop safety systems to help themselves and others. Some anxiety is essential to prepare for upcoming events, potential emergencies, or unexpected situations. It's what motivated people to follow safety

recommendations—such as using hand sanitizer, wearing a mask, and practicing physical distancing—during the pandemic. The "don't worry; be happy" people die the earliest from accidents and preventable illnesses.[7] Think of the people who were crowding the beaches during spring break in Florida when the coronavirus was beginning to spread in the United States.

My wife, Tana, grew up with these dragons. Her life was unpredictable and often scary. One of her first memories was her mother and grandmother falling to the floor when they found out her uncle had been murdered in a drug deal gone wrong. Subsequently, she became a planner and prepared for the worst. One might call her a prepper, which used to irritate me, but when the global pandemic hit, she was prepared, and never again will I say something when she tries to prepare for the end of the world.

3. **Strategies:** These will help you retrain and calm your emotional brain.

**Diaphragmatic breathing in a very specific pattern:**

1. Inhale for three seconds through your nose.
2. Hold for one second.
3. Exhale for six seconds (twice as long as inhale).
4. Hold for one second.
5. Repeat 10 times.
6. This will take less than two minutes.

When someone gets upset, angry, or anxious, his or her breathing becomes shallow and fast. This causes a change in the oxygen level in the anxious person's blood, making him or her more anxious. It becomes a vicious cycle, causing irritability, impulsiveness, confusion, and bad decision-making.

Learning to direct and control your breathing has immediate benefits. It calms the amygdala, counteracts the body's fight-or-flight response, relaxes muscles, warms hands, and regulates heart rhythms. I often teach patients to become experts at this breathing pattern, breathing slowly, deeply, and from their bellies. If you watch a baby or a puppy breathe, you will notice that they breathe almost solely with their bellies—the most efficient way to breathe. Expanding your belly when you inhale increases the amount of air available to your lungs and body. Pulling your belly in when you exhale causes the diaphragm to push the air out of your lungs, allowing for a more fully exhaled breath, which once again encourages deep breathing.

**Prayer and meditation** can calm the amygdala. A 2009 study in the *International Journal of Psychiatry in Medicine* found that prayer may be useful in the treatment of anxiety and depression.[8] I have performed several studies showing how meditation can calm the emotional brain and strengthen your prefrontal cortex, which I call the Dragon Tamer (you'll learn more about the Dragon Tamer in section 7). Meditation is a mental exercise in which you focus your attention on a specific thought, object, or activity for a short period of time. One of my favorite forms of meditation is called loving-kindness meditation, which is intended to develop feelings of goodwill and warmth toward others. It quickly increases positive emotions and decreases negative ones,[9] decreases pain[10] and migraine headaches,[11] reduces symptoms of post-traumatic stress disorder (PTSD)[12] and social prejudice,[13] increases gray matter in the emotional processing areas of the brain,[14] and boosts social connectedness.[15] Here's how to do it:

**Loving-kindness meditation:** Sit in a comfortable and relaxed position and close your eyes. Take two or three deep breaths, taking twice as long to exhale. Let any worries or concerns drift away, and feel your breath moving through the area around your heart. As you sit, quietly or silently repeat the following or similar phrases:

May I be safe and secure.
May I be healthy and strong.
May I be happy and purposeful.
May I be at peace.

Let the intentions in these phrases sink in as you repeat them. Allow the feelings to grow deeper. After a few repetitions, direct the phrases to someone you feel grateful for:

May you be safe and secure.
May you be healthy and strong.
May you be happy and purposeful.
May you be at peace.

Next visualize someone you feel neutral about. Choose among

people you neither like nor dislike, and repeat the phrases. Then visualize someone you don't like or with whom you are having a hard time. Kids who are being teased or bullied at school often feel quite empowered when they send love to the people who are making them miserable. Finally, direct the phrases toward everyone universally: "May all beings be safe and secure." You can do this for a few minutes or longer; it's up to you.

**Hypnosis** is a powerful tool to help gain control over your mind. Many people associate hypnosis with loss of control or stage tricks, but Stanford University psychiatrist David Spiegel writes that hypnosis is "a very powerful means of changing the way we use our minds to control perception and our bodies."[16] Learning hypnosis and similar techniques, such as guided imagery and progressive muscle relaxation, involves heightening focus and attention to enter a trancelike state that will help you relax. There are many online resources that can guide you, and we have several audios on our Brain Fit Life site (mybrainfitlife.com).

**Use your five senses to calm your emotional brain.** The brain senses the world. If you can change the inputs, you can often quickly change how you feel.

Vision—look at images of nature; create a folder of images that make you feel happy.

Hearing—develop a playlist of soothing music, such as David Lanz's "Beloved."

Touch—get a hug, massage, acupressure, or sit in a sauna for better touch inputs.

Smell—inhale calming scents, such as lemon, lavender, honeysuckle, rose, jasmine, or vanilla.

Tastes—savor chocolate, cinnamon, saffron, mint, nutmeg.

4. **Affirmations to say or meditate on every day:**

I am safe.

I am secure.

I am calm.

I am protected.

I focus on my breathing and centering myself.

# WOUNDED DRAGONS

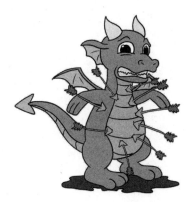

**Origin:** You experienced trauma, such as physical, emotional, or sexual abuse, or intense stress, such as being taken into foster care or being in a fire, flood, or assault. Bullying and being teased can also develop these dragons. The coronavirus pandemic traumatized nearly everyone on the planet, effectively creating a new army of Wounded Dragons around the world.

**Triggers:** Anything that remotely reminds you of the past trauma, including the smells, sights, sounds, and dates, such as an anniversary of the accident, death, divorce, breakup, or firing. In the future, these things may bring up memories of the pain you experienced.

When I was in high school, Cat Stevens was one of my favorite singer-songwriters. "Father and Son," "Moonshadow," "Peace Train," "Wild World," "Hard Headed Woman," "Morning Has Broken," and many more of his songs are etched into the tracks of my brain and attached to a happy time in my life. At the time, my wife, Tana, was a young child being raised in a home where her uncle was a drug addict. He and his drug addict friends also liked Cat Stevens, and she associated his music with an anxious, unpredictable time in her life. Fifty years later, whenever I play Cat Stevens, it brings joy to me, but it makes her angry and irritated. It triggers her Wounded Dragons and transforms them into angry ones.

**Reactions:** These dragons often cause people to relive trauma, have flashbacks and nightmares, feel numb, avoid situations that remind them of the event, feel that their future is short, always watch for bad things to happen, and panic when events remotely resemble an upsetting one from the past. People expend energy avoiding thoughts or feelings associated with a past

trauma. The following symptoms are common for those with Wounded
Dragons:

Recurrent and upsetting thoughts of a past traumatic event (pandemic
   lockdown, molestation, accident, fire, etc.)
Recurrent distressing dreams of a past upsetting event
Persistent avoidance of activities/situations that cause remembrance
   of upsetting event
Inability to recall an important aspect of a past upsetting event
Marked decreased interest in important activities
Feelings of detachment or distance from others
Numbness or restricted feelings
Instances of being startled easily
Marked physical response to events that are reminders of a past
   upsetting event, such as sweating when getting in a car because of a
   past car accident

**Movies:** These dragons are drawn to movies about healing, such as *Good Will Hunting*, *A Beautiful Mind*, *The Lion King*, *Ray*, and *As Good as It Gets*.

**Daniel's Wounded Dragons:** When I was young, we had a beautiful white goat named Sugar. All the kids adored her, but Sugar loved eating the bark off my father's trees. One day my late father had enough of Sugar damaging his prized plants and sent her away, which devastated us. At dinner a few days later, we learned that one of our uncles had slaughtered Sugar, and he joked that we were eating Sugar shish kebabs. I remembered it during one of my own therapy sessions many years later and cried for a long time. It was clearly traumatic.

*Tools to tame your Wounded Dragons*

1. **Do you recognize Wounded Dragons in your life?** Have you experienced trauma?

2. **Find the upside:** If you remember the pain and trauma from the
   past, it can help you break it for future generations; if, however, you
   repress it, you are more likely to repeat it. One of my friends, UFC
   fighter Justin Wren, who was bullied as a child and struggled with
   addiction and depression, found meaning and purpose in his life
   by starting a foundation called Fight for the Forgotten, which aims

to empower people worldwide who have been bullied or forgotten. Among many accomplishments, the foundation has helped 1,500 formerly enslaved pygmies in the jungles of the Congo gain their freedom and take ownership of 3,000 acres of land with access to clean water and farms.

When a trauma causes you to become stronger, it is called post-traumatic growth (PTG). I coined the term *post-pandemic growth* for those who have become stronger from the coronavirus outbreak. PTG happens in about 10 percent of people who experience traumas and includes a deepened spiritual life, a new appreciation of life, a vision for new possibilities, a positive change in relationships, and an increase in personal strength (*If I can survive this, I can survive most things*).

## 3. Strategies:

**Know when your nervous system is out of balance and bring it back.** Trauma tends to activate our sympathetic nervous system (SNS), the fight-or-flight response that makes us feel anxious and afraid. In a healthy nervous system, our parasympathetic nervous system (PNS) counterbalances the SNS and helps us calm down. They work in concert to help us manage stress.

When trauma is severe or prolonged, as it is in a months-long pandemic, the SNS can be "stuck on," making people feel anxious, panicked, hyperaroused, hypervigilant, restless, and sleepless, and have diarrhea. Or it can be "stuck off," leaving people feeling depressed, flat, exhausted, confused, and disoriented.

Recognize where your nervous system is. If it is stuck on, calm it with meditation, prayer, hypnosis, guided imagery, diaphragmatic breathing, and calming supplements, such as GABA, magnesium, or theanine. If it is stuck off, activate it with physical exercise, such as dancing or table tennis.

**Try trauma-focused cognitive behavioral therapy (TF-CBT).** Developed in the 1990s by a trio of professionals,[17] TF-CBT can be effective for children, teenagers, and adults who have experienced trauma. This therapy aims to help trauma survivors overcome anxiety, depression, guilt, anger, powerlessness, self-abuse, and acting out. In some ways it is similar to the ANT therapy you will read about in section 3. To find a TF-CBT therapist, visit tfcbt.org.

**Put your story on paper, and tell both sides.** Writing the story of your life in a balanced way that includes not only the traumas you have experienced but also the happy moments can be beneficial in coping with past hurts. This unique therapy, which is called narrative exposure therapy, encourages you to relive the emotions of the events while remaining rooted in the present. Multiple studies show this psychotherapy for trauma can be effective.[18] For more information, check out the narrative exposure therapy channel on the Vivo International website (vivo.org).

**Stop avoiding the pain from past trauma.** It's okay to experience painful feelings and emotions related to experiences that hurt you. Trying to stuff down or block your emotions can backfire. A wealth of research shows that avoidance raises the risk of psychological problems, including PTSD,[19] depression,[20] anxiety disorders,[21] and more. In those moments when you are suffering, reach out to a friend or therapist you can talk to, or write out what you are feeling.

**Break the bonds of the past.** A powerful technique I use with patients who struggle with Wounded Dragons is something I call breaking the bonds of the past. It is a way to help you reframe and disconnect from past memories. Whenever your Wounded Dragons whisper painful memories inside your head, answer the following questions on a piece of paper:

1. When was the last time you struggled, had the painful or disruptive memory or feeling, or felt suffering? Write down the details.

2. What were you feeling at the time? Describe the predominant feeling.

3. When was the first time you had that feeling? In your mind, imagine yourself on a train going backward through time. Go back to the time when you first had the feeling. Write down the incident or incidents in detail.

4. Can you go back even further to a time when you had that original feeling? Write down the details of the original incident.

5. If you have a clear idea of the origins of the feelings, can you disconnect them by reprocessing them through an adult or parent mindset, or reframe them in light of new information? Consciously disconnect the emotional bridge to the past with the idea that what happened in the past belongs in the past, and what happens now is what matters.

This is the technique I wrote about in the Introduction, where Jimmy remembered the origin of his fear of public speaking.

---

*Write out the story of the hurts from the past, see it from your adult perspective, and work to re-parent or soothe your inner child.*

---

**Consider eye movement desensitization and reprocessing (EMDR).** This form of psychotherapy can be helpful to eliminate or decrease the pain from past wounds and traumas. It is one of the most effective tools for quieting trauma. Traumatic events can get stuck in the brain's emotional centers and prevent it from processing information as it normally does. Then when someone recalls the trauma, the memory triggers an intense reexperiencing of the original event, complete with all its upsetting sights, sounds, smells, thoughts, and feelings. In this treatment, therapists have their clients think about the trauma and then direct their eye movements to go from side to side for a period of time (or they do alternate tapping on knees or arms). This alternate hemisphere brain stimulation has a calming effect on the brain.[22] Karen Lansing and I did a study on police officers who were involved in shootings and could no longer work. Their emotional brains were "stuck on." After an average of eight EMDR sessions, all of our officers went back to work, and this part of their emotional brains was significantly calmer.[23]

---

*See emdria.org to find an EMDR therapist near you.*

---

**EXAMPLE OF BEFORE AND AFTER EMDR, ACTIVE SPECT SCANS**

Before treatment                                                          After treatment

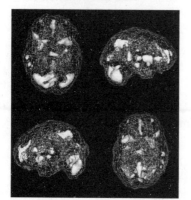 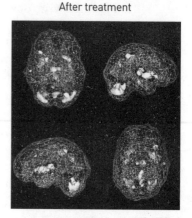

Diamond pattern of emotional activation
(white represents areas of highest activity)

Overall calming

**Wrap up in a weighted blanket.** Sleep issues are common in people who have been wounded. Research suggests that using a weighted blanket, which simulates being held or hugged safely and firmly, can assist in reducing anxiety and insomnia.[24]

4. **Affirmations to say or meditate on every day:**

I am safe in this moment.
I have everything I need in this moment.
That was then; this is now.
I release trauma, turmoil, and grief.
Asking for help is a sign of strength.

## SHOULD AND SHAMING DRAGONS

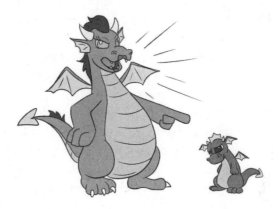

**Origin:** You were raised in a culture of guilt; you were humiliated, embarrassed, belittled, judged, or criticized. This happens in many religions and cultures with strong moral teachings, rules, and laws; shame can be a strong motivator to get people to comply.

**Triggers:** Disapproval from someone important to you, such as a parent, spouse, boss, coworker, or leader; perceived disapproval from God.

**Reactions:** These dragons can cause you to feel guilty, foolish, distressed, exposed, overly sensitive, or submissive, and they can make you want to hide, withdraw, or engage in self-harmful behaviors in secret, such as addictions, pornography, and overeating, which become dragons in their own right (see sections 4 and 6). They can also be the seeds of anxiety, depression, and obsessive thinking.

**Movies:** These dragons enjoy movies that poke fun at tradition, such as *M*A*S*H, The Help*, or *Meet the Parents*.

**Daniel's Should and Shaming Dragons:** Besides the Anxious Dragons, the bedwetting also activated my Should and Shaming Dragons. But it was not the only source. Once, when I was six or seven, I told my mother a lie. I have no idea what it was about, but I remember my mother started crying when she discovered it and told me, "I never thought I would have a son who was going to hell." She was usually more encouraging, but that moment stuck with me for a long time.

Growing up, my father called me a maverick, which to him was not a good thing, because I didn't just go along with all of his commands and wishes.

I was an inquisitive child who asked why and questioned him whenever I had a thought different from his. A fun fact I later learned was that my father was also labeled a maverick by many of the people in the grocery industry.

The Should and Shaming Dragons caused me to stay in a marriage that was not happy or healthy for 20 years, when I knew after a year it would never be great. I could not bring myself to deal with the shame of divorce that was taught in my culture and religion.

However, the maverick part of me served me well in another area. As I saw flaws in my profession as a psychiatrist, I worked hard to develop a new way of thinking. Yes, this invited vitriol from my colleagues, but being beaten up by my brother when I was young and standing up to my father helped me deal with the negative professional onslaught and push forward to do something special in my life.

### Tools to tame your Should and Shaming Dragons

1. **Do you recognize Should and Shaming Dragons in your life?** Do you routinely feel like guilt is motivating your actions and prompting you to do things that don't fit in with your values? Does shame prevent you from living the life you want?

2. **Find the upside:** Of course, there are things you should and should not do. Morality is essential for the greater good. That's why we have rules and laws. Shame and guilt can be helpful if these emotions serve your life goals; they can be hurtful if they make you feel bad, small, or disconnected from others.

   Shame can motivate learning, growth, and a desire to change and be better. It can help us lose weight and overcome an addiction; it can also help maintain social order, for without shame, people may engage in shameless acts. Shame can motivate us to reconnect and reconcile with others. It can inform and protect us from acting on impulses to engage in unhealthy behavior.

3. **Strategies:**

   **Break up with guilt.** Know when "should" and shame are helpful and when they are not. Do these thoughts or emotions serve you by helping you change something harmful in your life, or do they hurt you, causing you to feel like you're bad, evil, or a failure? If they do not serve you, break up with them. During the later years of my father's life, I would think, *I should go see my dad.* But thinking *I should* just made me feel bad. Trying to motivate yourself through guilt isn't helpful. I teach my patients to replace the word *should* with "It's my goal to" or "I want to" to see if the behavior still fits. For example, if you often think, *I should finish this presentation for work,* change the thought to, *I want to finish this presentation for work because it will help me get the promotion I want.* This will make you more motivated to do it. On the other hand, if an activity doesn't fit into your overall goals, you may feel more empowered by striking it from your to-do list. I started saying, "I want to see my dad," and it prompted me to visit him more often. Now that he's gone, I'm so grateful for that time we spent together.

**Realize the past is the past.** Behavior is much more complicated than most people think. We all make mistakes. It's part of learning and growing. Let your mistakes teach you something useful rather than tear you down. Then move forward.

**Revisit your childhood** to see if the origins for these dragons make sense or were used by others to control your thinking or behavior. See your younger self with love and compassion. How would a loving parent treat him or her? That is the best way to work on treating yourself.

**Reflect on what triggers the feelings of shame.** Common triggers include constructive criticism at school or work, sermons, lectures from your parents, a harsh comment from your significant other, a disapproving look from your mother-in-law when she tastes the food you've prepared for a family dinner, and more. Whenever you feel shame, close your eyes and imagine the first time you ever had that feeling to see if the events are connected.

**Talk to someone about the shame you feel.** Hiding from it expands it. Facing it takes away its power. Sharing these thoughts gets them out of your head and can help your brain move forward while leaving shame behind.

**Practice forgiveness for yourself and others.** On page 53, I include tips for forgiveness. Sometimes forgiving yourself can be harder than forgiving others. Try to show yourself the same kindness and compassion you would extend to others.

4. **Affirmations to say or meditate on every day:**

Each day I feel more at peace with my past mistakes.
I work to learn the lessons of my past.
I can and will let go of any shame that haunts me.
I replace *I should do this* with *Does it fit my overall goals to do this?*
That was then; this is now.

# SPECIAL, SPOILED, OR ENTITLED DRAGONS

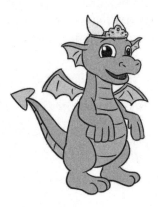

**Origin:** These are the "special" dragons, the golden children, and the miracle babies. Sometimes it is the oldest child, youngest child, or only child. Your parents wanted and loved you so much that they could never tell you no and treated you as the anointed or favored one who could do nothing wrong. They may still treat you this way. Your caregivers never wanted you to experience any pain, so they did everything for you, sometimes even your homework. You ended up with an artificially elevated sense of entitlement. I also see this type in some of the young musicians or actors I've treated. They were famous at a young age and felt as though they were special (they were), but it didn't serve their development.

**Triggers:** When you don't get your way; when others try to make you take responsibility; or when you don't feel as though you are treated as special.

**Reactions:** Lack of empathy for others, thinking others don't matter much and they are easy to cut off; tantrums, anger, rudeness, a strong need for attention, or a sense of injustice and outrage. You often say, "You owe me . . . ," "I deserve . . . ," or "It's their fault . . ."

**Movies:** These dragons love movies like *The Wolf of Wall Street*, *Catch Me If You Can*, *The Devil Wears Prada*, *Cruel Intentions*, *Mean Girls*, and *10 Things I Hate About You*.

**Daniel's Special, Spoiled, or Entitled Dragons:** I was the third of seven children, so these were not my dragons. I was, however, named after my grandfather, who was my best friend growing up. He made me feel very special.

Years later, after becoming a physician and bestselling author, I did have times when I was too full of myself and reacted negatively at work or home when I did not get what I thought I deserved. This is where your Should and Shaming Dragons can keep the Special, Spoiled, or Entitled Dragons under control.

---

*I define entitlement as two beliefs:*
*(1) I am exempt from responsibility; and*
*(2) I am owed special treatment. These beliefs*
*cause alienation and frustration and are ultimately*
*destructive to the future of the entitled person.*

**DR. JOHN TOWNSEND**

---

### Tools to tame your Special, Spoiled, or Entitled Dragons

1. **Do you recognize Special, Spoiled, or Entitled Dragons in your life?** Do you regularly expect to be the center of attention, feel like others should do things for you, and think that many everyday activities are beneath you?

2. **Find the upside:** Feeling special and having a cheering section helps your self-esteem, as long as it doesn't hurt others.

3. **Strategies:**

   **Take responsibility for your life.** Responsibility is not about fault but, rather, your ability to respond. Change the phrase "I deserve . . ." to "I am responsible for . . ."

   **Notice how good it feels to promote the success of other people.**

   **Practice seeing things from another person's point of view.**

Catch yourself justifying your spoiled actions.

Spend less time around people who act entitled.

4. Affirmations to say or meditate on every day:

I am special, but so is everyone around me.
I am responsible for my own happiness.
I encourage the success of others.
I see things from the other person's point of view.
Acting spoiled spoils my own happiness and joy.

# RESPONSIBLE DRAGONS

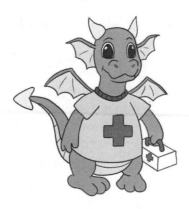

**Origin:** You feel liable for the pain or situation of others, often because you felt powerless to help someone you cared about, such as a parent or sibling who was suffering. This became rampant during the onset of the pandemic when hospitals would not allow family members to visit sick or dying loved ones. Or you felt insignificant, and fixing other people's issues helped you feel significant. Children believe they are at the center of the universe, so if something good happens they think it's because of them; but if something bad happens to someone they love, they often think it is because of them and feel responsible, even though their thinking is irrational.

The eldest child in a family often feels a natural sense of responsibility toward younger siblings, and neglectful parents sometimes task older children with taking care of the younger kids even though they are not emotionally equipped to handle the responsibility. During the early months of the coronavirus pandemic, due to school closures, many tweens and teens had to assume adult responsibilities at home if parents were still going to work. They will likely develop Responsible Dragons that need taming.

**Triggers:** When you perceive others in need.

**Reactions:** This fixer, caretaker, codependent dragon can cause you to do too much for others, so they become dependent on you, which ultimately breeds entitlement and resentment, and creates unbalanced relationships and long-term stress.

**Movies:** These dragons love movies about healers, such as *Awakenings*, *Ordinary People*, *The Doctor*, and *Patch Adams*.

**Daniel's Responsible Dragons:** When I became an infantry medic at the age of 18, I discovered a sense of significance (it helped to tame my Insignificant Dragons). As I felt responsible for the well-being of others, over time I realized if I do too much, it can create an unnecessary dependency, increasing everyone's stress. My wife, Tana, says I want to save the world. When our nieces went into foster care five years ago at a time when Tana was estranged from her half-sister, I knew we had to act. My Responsible Dragons made me feel very uncomfortable. I was horrified with the idea of children away from their parents, scared, alone and feeling unloved, even though I did not know these nieces. It caused tension between Tana and me because she had purposely distanced herself from that part of her family as a result of their poor judgment and behavior. We eventually figured out solutions together to help the parents get healthier, and the children now live with us, which brings us joy.

### Tools to tame your Responsible Dragons

1. **Do you recognize Responsible Dragons in your life?** Do you tend to take on too much responsibility?

2. **Find the upside:** There is a lot of upside for Responsible Dragons. You get to help, be in charge, and have others in your debt. You also get to be part of a community you are creating. Good deeds reduce physical pain.[25] Helping others is altruistic and helps you.

3. **Strategies:**

   **Realize that doing too much for others can create dependency and inhibit them from being independent and self-sufficient.** It's a balancing act between being helpful and teaching others to be competent on their own.

   **Self-care is not selfish.** Remember what they say on airplanes, "If the masks come down, put yours on first." Prioritize taking care of yourself to the same degree that you care for others. This includes setting healthy boundaries. You're limited and need to accept those limitations; otherwise, you burn out, max out, and fizzle out. If you don't, it's easy to resent those you help, seeing them as needy and taking, taking, taking all the time.

**Evaluate the people in your life.** In his book *People Fuel*, Dr. John Townsend lists seven types of people in your life:

1. Coaches (mentors)
2. Comrades (very close friends and loved ones)
3. Casuals (friends)
4. Colleagues (coworkers)
5. Care (they depend on you)
6. Chronics (they always have issues)
7. Contaminants (they desire to damage others, controlled by their Angry Dragons)[26]

Do what you can to eliminate the Contaminant people and increase types 1–4. This is part of self-care and will bring better balance to your life.

Deal with your past responsibility for others. Try to identify the source of your Responsible Dragons and make peace with those experiences. You may need to work with a professional to help you come to terms with your past.

**4. Affirmations to say or meditate on every day:**

Loving others as myself means taking care of myself so I can love others.

I love helping others, as long as I'm helping them become competent and independent.

It is better to give than to receive, as long as giving does not create unnecessary dependency.

I share the load with others so I don't become overburdened or burned out.

I do what I can and trust others to God's care.

# ANGRY DRAGONS

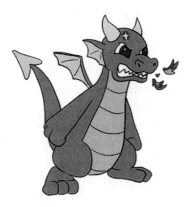

**Origin:** You were hurt, shamed, bullied, abused, disappointed, or perceived that you were hurt, shamed, or disappointed by others. Others modeled angry behavior for you. With stay-at-home orders due to the pandemic, many people experienced anger and frustration over things they could no longer do, or they were hurt financially. These frustrations and hurts may create new Angry Dragons.

**Triggers:** When anything reminds you of the hurts, shame, bullying, abusive behavior, or disappointments in the past; when others overwhelm you with words or want you to take responsibility for something.

**Reactions:** Irrational rage, frequent irritability, regular frustration, and rudeness or inconsiderate remarks. You may express your anger in actions, such as bullying, belittling, annoying, being disobedient, blaming, fighting, punishing, name-calling, or stonewalling. Common warning signs include heart rate increases, sweating, cold hands, muscle tension (especially in the neck), goose bumps, dizziness, or confusion.

**Movies:** Angry Dragons like horror movies that inflict fear and pain on others, such as *The Shining, Jaws, Halloween, The Texas Chainsaw Massacre,* and *Silence of the Lambs.*

**Daniel's Angry Dragons:** My father loved taking family videos during holidays. Until I was about six, most of them showed my brother pushing me down or hitting me. Being smaller and younger, I was at a disadvantage. By the time I was about seven, my brother realized I would be a better playmate than punching bag, and we started to do more together. But it set up the Angry Dragons in my life, looking out for someone who might try to hurt me and getting furious at those who tried to hurt others.

When George Floyd was killed by a police officer in May 2020 (nearly three months into the coronavirus restrictions), it fueled these dragons. In some people, the Angry Dragons were so powerful that they stomped all over their Anxious Dragons, inciting thousands across the nation and around the globe to disregard physical distancing—and for some to defy recommendations to wear a mask in public—in order to protest Floyd's death. It was as if all the fear of contracting COVID-19 was wiped from their brains when these Angry Dragons roared into action. This shows how your Dragons from the Past can battle each other for your attention.

### Tools to tame your Angry Dragons

1. **Do you recognize Angry Dragons in your life?** How often do you have any of the reactions listed above?

2. **Find the upside:** Anger can push us toward our goals, help us overcome obstacles, release steam, express feelings, and right wrongs (as long as we don't create more wrongs). Anger can be turned toward being assertive, creating energy, providing a sense of control, and making us aware of injustices.

   Angry people can be more optimistic. In one study, those who expressed anger in the aftermath of the 9/11 terrorist attacks expected fewer attacks in the future compared to those experiencing fear, who were more pessimistic.[27]

3. **Strategies:**

   **Make a list of 10 things to do when you are angry to distract yourself**, if only for a few minutes, to give your brain space to respond more appropriately, such as:

   1. Consciously focus on your goals for the situation.

   2. Be aware of your own danger signs before your anger is about to blow. When you feel these symptoms, take 10 deep breaths

(three seconds in; hold for one second; six seconds out; hold for one second), which takes less than two minutes. I can guarantee you will express your feelings in a more effective way afterward.

3. Take a time-out if you feel you cannot appropriately communicate or control yourself. This could mean leaving the house, hanging up the phone, or rescheduling a meeting.

4. Listen to soothing music.

5. Take a walk or exercise to release some of the excessive energy.

6. Take a shower or bath to wash off the negative feelings.

7. Journal your negative thoughts to get them out of your head and evaluate them (see the ANTs section on page 97).

8. Keep a lavender sachet and inhale the aroma with five deep breaths when upset.

9. Eat a healthy snack in case you are hangry because your blood sugar is low.

10. Take a brief nap in case you are sleep deprived.

**Anger can be good if it is directed positively and appropriately for present-day reasons.** When you feel anger, ask yourself if the problem really is now or from a time long past. If it is from the past, work to express that anger in a safe, controlled way. If possible, direct it to the person or people who originally caused the issues, so you can make peace with them and shed the pent-up anger. This process may require the help of a mental health professional. If it is something to deal with now, after you've calmed yourself, brainstorm ways to constructively express your concerns.

**Know when to seek help.** Sometimes anger comes from brain systems that have been hurt or are dysfunctional. If you've calmed yourself physically and assessed that your anger is not in relation to a current situation within your realm to address, then you may benefit from brain imaging to determine if undetected brain issues, such as a hidden traumatic brain injury, problems in the temporal lobes, or sleepy frontal lobes may be contributing to anger issues.

4. **Affirmations to say or meditate on every day:**

I express my anger in ways so that others can hear.
I accept responsibility if my anger has hurt someone.
I direct my anger appropriately.
I do not use anger to scare or frighten other people.
I express my anger in words, never physical actions, unless
    someone I love is threatened.

## JUDGMENTAL DRAGONS

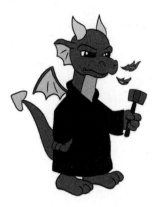

**Origin:** You grew up in an environment where you were hurt or perceived life as unfair. People played favorites, were inconsistent in how they applied rules, and may have left you out of activities and important decisions.

**Triggers:** Whenever you feel injustice to yourself, or others, or when you see others doing something you think is wrong. In the first few months of the pandemic, Judgmental Dragons seemed to breathe fire over the entire world, causing people to quickly judge others for their actions (wearing a mask or not wearing a mask, etc.). Then after these Judgmental Dragons had already been let loose, the death of George Floyd caused them to run wild. Many people unfairly judged all police officers based on the actions of the few involved in Floyd's death. Others made blanket judgments about protestors, blaming all of them for the rioting, looting, and mayhem that took place, even though most had protested peacefully.

**Reactions:** Condescending, criticizing, moralizing, correcting people, or telling others what they should and should not think or do.

**Movies:** These dragons love vengeance movies, such as the Rambo and Taken series, and especially *Law Abiding Citizen*.

**Daniel's Judgmental Dragons:** I'm the third of seven children, so competing for attention and significance, as well as issues of fairness and judgment, have always been part of my psyche. As an adult, I've spent three decades trying to improve my psychiatric profession by adding brain imaging tools and natural ways to heal the brain. In doing so, I have received a lot of criticism, which has brought forth my Judgmental Dragons as a response, and I can be harsher on my colleagues than is helpful.

My wife, Tana, has these dragons as well. When we first met, she had very strong opinions on criminal behavior, especially about drug addicts and child molesters, and she could come across as the judge, jury, and executioner. Knowing that I had testified in death penalty murder trials for the defense made her wonder about my sanity. Her attitude was understandable since she grew up in an unsafe environment with an uncle who was a heroin addict. Her stepfather also molested her. Over time, as she understood our brain imaging work, her heart softened, and the Judgmental Dragons became more balanced. She still thinks all child molesters should die, even though she is more willing to listen to the evidence.

When Larry King was at CNN, his producer called me to help with a show they were doing about a gang rape in the Bay Area. They wanted me to talk about my brain imaging work with criminals. I had to drive from my office in Orange County to Hollywood to be at the studio at 5 p.m. Since Los Angeles traffic is rated as among the world's worst, I asked Tana to go with me so I could use the car-pool lane. When she found out why I was appearing on Larry's show, her Judgmental Dragons breathed fire on me the whole drive there and back.

### Tools to tame your Judgmental Dragons

1. **Do you recognize Judgmental Dragons in your life?** Do you tend to make snap judgments about others?

2. **Find the upside:** These dragons can help you feel in control and clarify your values and goals. They also want to right wrongs and protect those who are victims. They can guide your actions and help you make pro-social choices. Like anger, judgment can be good if it is directed positively for present-day reasons.

3. **Strategies:**

   **Ask a few questions when you feel judgmental.** Is the problem now, or are you trying to right a wrong from the past? Do you have all the facts, or are you making assumptions about others that you do not know are true?

**REACH for forgiveness.** Psychologist Everett Worthington of Virginia Commonwealth University has studied forgiveness for years and developed a model for forgiveness called REACH,[28] which stands for:

Recall the hurt—This time recall it differently, without feeling victimized or holding a grudge. This moves you toward relating to the offense from the point of view of the offender.

Empathize—Replace negative emotions with positive, others-oriented emotions. This involves putting yourself in the shoes of the person who hurt you and imagining what he/she might have been feeling.

Altruism—Give the gift of your forgiveness to the person who hurt you. Think about a time in your past when you wronged someone and that person forgave you, and remember how much freer you felt. That is your gift.

Commit to the forgiveness that you experience—making a public statement of your forgiveness shapes your internal reality. Cement your feelings by engaging in a ritual like completing a forgiveness certificate or writing a word that symbolizes the offense on your hand and then washing it off.

Hold on to the forgiveness—If/when you encounter the offender, you may feel anger and fear, and you may worry that you haven't really forgiven him or her. That is just your body's response as a warning to be careful, not a lack of forgiveness.

In 1996, Dr. Worthington's research was put to the worst possible test: His mother was murdered in a home invasion. Although police believed they had found the murderer, he was never prosecuted. Despite the awful tragedy, Dr. Worthington said, "I had applied the forgiveness model many times, but never to such a big event. As it turned out, I was able to forgive the young man quite quickly."[29]

Apply Worthington's model to yourself. Tana tells a story about her involvement in a brain health program we were asked to develop for the Salvation Army's largest chemical addiction recovery program. After her first visit to the campus, she was suddenly filled with highly judgmental thoughts about the addicts in the program. It's clear that clean eating helps people with addictions make better decisions, so she wanted to participate. But how could she help people who brought up feelings of fear and loathing inside her? Most of the participants (beneficiaries) are court ordered to the program, and many go there after having served time in jail for some serious criminal offenses.

Growing up, Tana directly experienced the consequences that drugs can have on people's lives. As mentioned above, her uncle was murdered in a drug deal gone wrong. She hated drugs and had no tolerance for anyone who did them. When she told me she didn't think she could follow through with helping at the Salvation Army, that God had picked the wrong person this time, I smiled and said, "God picked the perfect person." In fact, working with that population gave Tana new empathy for their backgrounds, which were not that much different from her own. And she realized that for every person she helped, there would be one less scared child in the world. REACH for forgiveness helped to tame her Judgmental Dragons.

**Be curious, not furious.** When you find yourself making a snap judgment about others, ask what might be behind their behavior. Are they having a bad day? Did they just get laid off from work? Did they just find out a loved one has cancer? Do they live in a chaotic environment filled with chronic stress? It's easy to say people are jerks, rude, or inconsiderate; it's harder to ask why.

**Are you actually feeling insecure?** It's possible that you criticize others as a way to feel better about yourself. So if you find yourself denigrating others for their successes, for example, recognize these thoughts as envy. Then reframe these negative thoughts to focus on being proud of what you have accomplished in life without comparing yourself to others.

**Judge behaviors, not people.** Does one mistake make someone a bad person? We've all done something stupid, and none of us would like to be judged solely on our worst moment or our worst day. Try to step back to view a person's overall qualities, not just their faults or particular actions.

**Get out of your bubble.** If you're quick to judge others, it may be due to unfamiliarity with others outside your immediate social circle.

Experience new settings, and meet people who have different experiences from you as a way to enhance your understanding and empathy. This can help you embrace the differences among people rather than judge them.

4. **Affirmations to say or meditate on every day:**

I trade judgment for understanding.
I release judgment so I can feel free.
I treat people in pain with compassion, not more pain.
I am a role model for what I want to see in the world.
I foster peace in this situation so there will be more peace
    in the world.

## DEATH DRAGONS

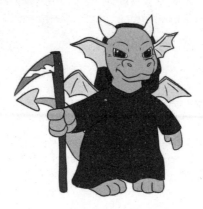

**Origin:** These dragons are always with us and often rear their heads during midlife—when your spouse leaves you for a younger person, when you have a health scare, when you start having trouble performing in the bedroom, when your parents or your friends' parents die and you start going to funerals. You wonder if this is all there is to life, hence a midlife crisis. They can start earlier if you have to confront death because of living during a pandemic, being in an accident, being diagnosed with a life-threatening illness such as cancer, having a friend from high school die by suicide, or having a parent or sibling with a serious illness. Fear of aging, getting old, or losing your youth; feeling that your life is not meaningful; or fearing others will not survive or thrive without you also provide the energy for these dragons.

When the global pandemic upended our lives, it fired up the Death Dragons and led to premature midlife crises. People in their twenties and thirties were suddenly deciding to make a major "career pivot" away from the corporate ladder and toward something more meaningful to them. A BBC News article featured young adults who were turning their backs on their career paths and embracing new work based on what they were truly passionate about—painting or embroidery, for example.[30] During the pandemic, I often imagined the Death Dragons as Godzilla, breathing fire as he scorched the population of the earth.

**Triggers:** Pandemics, illnesses, funerals, near-miss accidents, losing friends or loved ones, looking in the mirror and seeing wrinkles or other signs of aging.

**Reactions:** A pervading sense of doom, panic attacks, or fear of aging and dying can preoccupy your thoughts. These fears and anxieties can turn into physical illness, such as high blood pressure, heart disease, and gastrointestinal issues. These dragons can also lead to risky behaviors to test death.

**Movies:** These dragons love movies that offer hope about transformation and the afterlife, such as *Heaven Is for Real*, *Ghost*, and *The Five People You Meet in Heaven*. They also love movies that celebrate aging, such as *Harold and Maude*, *The Bucket List*, *Driving Miss Daisy*, *Cocoon*, and *On Golden Pond*.

**Daniel's Death Dragons:** Growing up in a religious home, the issues of death and the potential of an afterlife were always present. My mom's comment about me going to hell highlighted the issue earlier than was ideal. When I was an infantry medic, I drove an ambulance and got a close-up look at death for the first time, which weighed on me. In college I took a class called Death and Dying in which we studied death and I wrote my own obituary. It crystallized the fact that death is certainly coming for us all, but if we live as if we'll die, then we have more of an incentive to make the most of each day. My motivation to live a present, purposeful life was further strengthened when my grandfather and father passed away.

*Tools to tame your Death Dragons*

1. **Do you recognize Death Dragons in your life?** Are you filled with anxious thoughts about getting older, getting sick, or dying? Do you test death with risky behaviors?

2. **Find the upside:** Knowing you are going to die can help you live a meaningful life, plan for the future, and work to create a legacy. Cherishing each day can help you to resolve interpersonal conflicts and use listening skills and empathy, rather than stewing, ignoring issues, or holding a grudge.

3. **Strategies:**

   **Accept death as a natural part of life on this earth.** Psychiatrist Elisabeth Kübler-Ross, in her book *Death: The Final Stage of Growth*, wrote, "It is the denial of death that is partially responsible for people living empty, purposeless lives; for when you live as if you'll live forever, it becomes too easy to postpone the things you know that you must do."[31]

**Create a list of what you want to accomplish during your life.** Be sure to make it meaningful. Choose activities that support your values and relationships.

**Focus on issues that have eternal value** (after you've taken care of today by taking care of your health and supporting your family), meaning they have value beyond today and support God's purposes for your life. I frequently ask myself, *Does this issue have eternal value?* It helps me not sweat the small stuff, and over time I've realized that most things are the small stuff.

**List good things about dying.** Here are some of mine:

- My faith leads me to believe I will have eternal life.
- I may get to see my father and grandfather again.
- No more people coughing on airplanes.
- No more traffic. I live near Los Angeles, so this is a big deal.
- No more internet trolls.
- No more divisive political campaigns, at least I hope not.
- No more taxes.
- No more spam or junk mail.
- I won't have to shave anymore and deal with the occasional cuts and bleeding.
- I won't have to get my teeth cleaned and have someone with a sharp metal object poking around my mouth.
- No more root canals.
- No more computer crashes where I lose an hour's worth of work.

4. **Affirmations to say or meditate on every day:**

I will live a life that matters.
I will live life fully and fearlessly.
I will be present today in all I do.
Death teaches me that if something is meaningful, I do it,
    but if it is not meaningful, I do not do it.
Death is just the next stage of eternal life.

## GRIEF AND LOSS DRAGONS

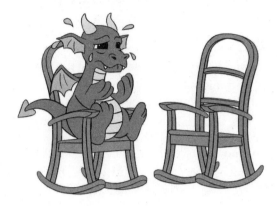

**Origin:** Grief and Loss Dragons are easy to find because they are everywhere, especially due to the coronavirus pandemic. These dragons show up as a reaction to losing *someone* important (death, separation and divorce, breakup of a love interest or close friendship or peer group, a partner to dementia, empty nest syndrome), *something* important (health—a mastectomy or an amputation, job, finances, beloved pet), or *an attachment to ideas* of what could have been (identity—retirement, loved one with an addiction, loss of success).

Any death—whether the expected loss of an elderly parent, the sudden death of a child, or the terminal illness of a pet—can trigger grief and loss. Death from suicide is particularly harsh because most people believe it was a simple choice when it was often the result of an invisible brain illness.

Over the years as a child psychiatrist, I've treated many parents who had autistic, learning disabled, or ADHD children. They often struggle with the grief of mourning what could have been and what they could have done differently to prevent the sorrow and pain. I've also treated a number of young superstar actors, musicians, and athletes. Sometimes they mourn the loss of their adolescence. They worked so hard then that they believe they missed out on the carefree, fun times. I remind them that few people really love their teenage years, so they were blessed to be able to work and succeed through it. It's a matter of perspective.

In the wake of the pandemic, nearly everyone experienced some form of loss—the death of a loved one from COVID-19, a career gone up in smoke, a graduation ceremony missed, a way of life interrupted, or a sense of freedom stolen.

**Triggers:** Anything that reminds you of the loss—a sight, a song, a routine (making coffee in the morning), anything. Whenever I see my mother at her home, memories of my father flood my brain.

**Reactions:** Shock, sadness, numbness, denial, despair, anger, guilt, loneliness, helplessness, yearning, anxiety, trouble breathing, chest pain, sleeplessness, or memory loss. Chronic stress shrinks the hippocampus, one of the major memory centers in the brain, and it suppresses the immune system, making you more vulnerable to infections and viruses such as COVID-19.

**Movies:** Inspiring movies shake these dragons out of their negative state and help them forget, such as *Soul Surfer, Chariots of Fire, Hacksaw Ridge, August Rush, The Sound of Music, Unbroken,* and *The Shawshank Redemption.*

**Daniel's Grief and Loss Dragons:** When you're 66, the age I am writing this, you've experienced plenty of grief and loss, whether divorce, children growing up and moving away, the end of other relationships or jobs, professional challenges, and more. The day my grandfather died was the worst single day of my life. I cried for a long time, and many years later whenever I think of him the tears just come, even as I write this. Once, 30 years after his death, I was on a trip with Tana shortly after we met, and there was terrible traffic on the freeway. We got off to take another route and happened to go by the cemetery where he was buried. When I realized his remains were just a few hundred yards away, I burst into tears and then spent the rest of the trip telling Tana about him. When my father died, it dredged up all those feelings about losing my grandfather.

### *Tools to tame your Grief and Loss Dragons*

1. **Do you recognize Grief and Loss Dragons in your life?** These are usually easy to spot, but often with a big loss, several smaller losses accompany it. For instance, if you lose a job, you also lose that income, some of your relationships at work, benefits, and future plans for yourself in that role.

2. **Find the upside:** After a loss, many people make health a priority. The joy I felt from my grandfather's love and the sadness I felt from losing him caused me to constantly ask myself two important questions over the last 40 years: (1) *How can I love other people like he loved me?* Isn't that really what life is about—being loving, connected, useful, and helpful? (2) *How can I take better care of my brain so that I*

*can love my family, be independent, and do the work I love for as long as possible?* After my father died, I felt even more motivated to dedicate my life to helping people achieve better brain health.

It's an opportunity to reset your deepest sense of meaning and purpose. My goal in becoming a psychiatrist was to be useful to those in need. It was never to be loved by my colleagues. Focusing on our work and ignoring those who don't appreciate it has been freeing.

Pain can open you up to be a comfort to others, as well as help you appreciate each moment and the important people in your life. Once, after the loss of an important relationship, one of my friends told me my heart was actually broken *open*. There was a strong truth to what she said. Part of you goes away when a loved one passes, but also a part of them stays. My grandfather and my father are always with me, and whenever I hold my five grandchildren, I also feel those two holding me.

## 3. Strategies:

**Start the healing process as soon as possible.** People may tell you to wait to heal from grief, but if you fell and broke your arm, when would you want to start healing? Immediately! This doesn't mean healing will be quick—it rarely is—but you start with one step. Dr. Kübler-Ross originally wrote about the five stages of grief: denial, anger, bargaining, depression, and acceptance. No matter what stage you're in, recognize it and start taking at least one of the following steps toward healing. To kick-start the healing process after my father died, I shared my grief with my social media followers with nightly live chats. It proved to be very cathartic for me, and I felt good about helping others navigate their feelings after the death of a loved one.

**Work to turn the five stages of grief upside down.** Rather than denial, anger, bargaining, depression, and acceptance, admit your loss, find peace, stop bargaining for something that will not change, reengage with others to avoid depression, and refuse to accept prolonged pain as a given.

**Keep a brain-healthy routine.** It's especially important to eat brain-healthy food, take supplements, exercise, and sleep. This is often the missing link in grief recovery. When people are in pain, they will often do nearly anything to stop it. Overeating, binge drinking, smoking marijuana, and other habits may put a temporary Band-Aid on the negative feelings but often prolong the pain.

**Fix sleep first.** Grief often steals sleep, so I often recommend a combination of melatonin (1 mg), vitamin B6 (10 mg), magnesium (100 mg), GABA (300 mg), 5-HTP (50 mg), and theanine (100 mg) to help promote grief-related sleep. If it is ineffective, I then try the medication trazodone in increasing doses. Insomnia decreases blood flow to the PFC in the front part of the brain. The PFC sends signals to quiet or calm your emotional brain; when it is weak, your emotions can get the best of you, and it is harder to make good decisions throughout the day.

**Consider supplements.** Loss and rejection are felt in the same part of the brain as physical pain. Supplements such as saffron, SAMe, curcumin, magnesium, and omega-3 fatty acids help physical pain and may also help emotional pain.

**Be on the alert for an ANT invasion**—especially the Guilt Beating and Blaming species (see section 3).

**Write out the story of what happened.** Spend 15 minutes a day for four days getting the story out, making sure to list both the positives ("He is no longer suffering") and the negatives ("I miss her so much it hurts") of the situation. Writing has helped refugee children and adolescents deal with grief,[32] and it has been shown to decrease feelings of loneliness and help improve mood.[33] In one study, bereaved people who had lost someone to an accidental death or homicide wrote for 15 minutes a day for four days. One group wrote about the loss; the other was asked to write about something trivial. Afterward, those who had written about the loss reported less anxiety and depression and greater grief recovery than those who had written about trivialities.[34] As you're writing, include anything that was left unsaid or unfinished. That way it will not endlessly spin in your mind. Talk to others about what you wish had been different so you can learn from it.

**Remember the positive; make peace with the rest.** Too often, people remember the good times and completely ignore the bad ones. Remembering an unbalanced situation prolongs grief. My grandmother was not that nice to my grandfather while he was alive, but she sainted him in death, which prolonged her grief. He really was a saint, but I resented that she didn't treat him that way when he was alive. I needed more forgiveness for her. When my dad died, my siblings gave me some grief because I admitted on social media chats that my father wasn't always a great dad. But I had to be honest about the relationship I had with him. I'm like most people who have conflicting feelings about the important people in their lives.

My dad was tough. One of his favorite sayings was "I don't get heart attacks; I give them." When I was growing up, my dad was so busy building a grocery store empire that he never had time to come to my games and rarely spent any alone time with me. As a teen when I was working for him, he fired me (that happened more than once), and he told a friend of mine I would never amount to anything. He later belittled me for wanting to be a "nut" doctor and never showed any respect for my professional accomplishments despite the success I had. It wasn't until he turned 85 that things changed. That was when he told me was tired of feeling sick—he had been suffering from health issues for some time—and asked me for help. That paved the way to the father-son bonding I had always yearned for. On the weekends, we would work out together, and in four months he lost 40 pounds and his health improved. From then on, I went from being the irritating and irritated second son to someone he relied on and trusted for medical advice. During those last five years of his life, he became one of my best friends, and I finally got the closeness I had wanted my whole life. I'm so grateful for that, and the memories of the past five years fill me with joy. I've made peace with all those years when he was too busy for me or was disrespectful to me.

**Remember that crying is normal.** After someone has died, it is healthy to let the tears flow freely. When we bottle our feelings and refuse to cry, our emotional brain becomes inflamed. When I was a resident at Walter Reed Medical Center in the eighties, I saw a colonel who had developed a rash all over his body. The dermatologist was stumped as to the cause and so was the internal medicine doctor.

It turned out the rash had started soon after his wife had unexpectedly died. As a hard-nosed army colonel, he didn't feel he could allow himself to cry. He thought he should just soldier on. Over the following year as I met with him, we broke down those beliefs, and he finally allowed himself to weep openly in front of me. After that, his rash went away.

**Reach out for social support.** Therapy and support groups can be beneficial if they help you build skills to overcome grief.

**Breathe with your belly.** When you get anxious or short of breath, belly breathing can calm you down or help you catch your breath.

**Get any chest pain checked out.** Chest pain is common in grief.[35] Stress hormones can make our hearts beat in an abnormal rhythm, which can cause chest pain. When I went through a period of grief, my chest hurt so badly I thought I had heart disease. I didn't. Likewise, after my assistant, Kim, lost her fiancé to a heart attack, she started to have chest pain too. When she had it evaluated, it turned out her coronary arteries were more than 90 percent blocked. She did have heart disease, which responded well to treatment. It turned out that the death of her fiancé may have saved her life. If you get chest pain, get a physical. If your heart is fine, practicing deep breathing, surrender prayers, guided imagery, and hypnosis can calm your brain, as can taking 250 mg of magnesium glycinate two to three times a day.

**Deal with triggers as they come up.** Getting triggered is particularly common in grief, especially when the person or pet can occupy every fun place in your brain. Whenever you get triggered by an anniversary, birthday, holiday, place, song, or smell, don't try to block the feeling; allow it to wash over you. Cry if tears flow, and allow yourself to be grateful for the memory. Don't avoid the feelings, and make sure to correct any negative thoughts that tag along with the painful feelings.

**Be patient. It is a journey, not a destination.** No one does grief perfectly. I lost someone important to me many years ago. I knew many of the right things to do, but I still suffered for several months and could not get the person out of my head. Ultimately, reading Byron Katie's book *Loving What Is*, which elegantly teaches you not to believe every stupid thought you have, was incredibly helpful. Be patient with yourself as you work through the hard times. Never forget, everyone in the family has their own dragons, and grief tends to trigger them. Be patient with others too.

**Honor your loved ones.** Use anniversaries to remember those you lost, not to suffer. Set a place for them at dinner, light a candle in their memory, or discuss the moments you loved with others. Soon after my father died, I wrote a poem to honor him and read at his memorial service, which we broadcast over Zoom because of the pandemic.

*Good Grief . . . he's everywhere in my brain.*

*I see him in every flower that blooms; he was a master gardener,*
*I see him in every brilliant Pacific sunset, which he loved to photograph repeatedly,*
*I see him every time we play cards and someone says gin; he was a master strategist who stomped us all,*
*I see him in his big chair surrounded by his grandchildren; he was a great, great grandfather,*
*I see him in every brain we scan, because he helped me invest in our first imaging cameras, and*
*I see him every time I check my Schwab account and look at the UNFI stock he recommended, which goes up and down like my emotions since he left.*

*Good Grief . . . he's everywhere in my brain.*

*I hear his beautiful deep voice saying, "Danny, it's your dad, give me a call. I have tangerines, avocados, and lemons." When I want to cry and have good grief, I play his voice mails over and over,*
*I hear him when the television blares too loud, because like me he has trouble hearing and won't wear hearing aids,*
*I hear him whenever someone says "bull----" or "no" or "I'm the boss, do what I say"; he was a very strong leader,*
*I hear him whenever I hear a tennis ball hit a racquet, as we had so many great games together.*

*I hear him when he tells me I can do anything I put my mind to; he
    encouraged so many people and set us all up for success.*

*Good Grief . . . he's everywhere in my brain.*

*I sense him whenever I smell a sweet orange from his ranch or a
    gardenia from his garden,*
*I sense him every time I go into a supermarket; it was his life,*
*I sense him every time someone calls me a maverick, because I inherited
    it from him,*
*I sense him whenever we go on vacation, because he taught us that
    families have fun together.*
*I sense him whenever our very large family gathers, which he and my
    mother created with love. When I told my mother that cinnamon
    was a natural aphrodisiac, she hit her forehead and said, "That's
    why we have seven children; he would never leave me alone."
    Lebanese cook with a lot of cinnamon.*

*Good Grief . . . he's everywhere in my brain.*

*I feel him every time I lift weights, as we did so many Sunday workouts
    together,*
*I feel him whenever I do a plank, knowing he would go longer than
    anyone in the room, even me, because he was so stubborn,*
*I feel him every time I walk Mr. Vinnie. I remember buying him for
    Dad because he was so sad when the original Vinnie died. He loved
    his dogs . . . sometimes more than his kids.*
*I feel him every time I remember kissing the top of his head when I'd say
    "See you next week," and*
*I'll always feel his soft hands before they took him away the day he died.*

*Good Grief . . . he's everywhere in my brain and is intricately woven
    into the fabric of my soul.*

*He was bold, brilliant, outspoken, and the essence of the American
Dream. I won't lie; early on it was hard being his son . . . the boss's kid.
How could anyone live up to the success he created? As a grocer he fed
thousands; he was a leader in his industry and a financial wizard. He
was tough, opinionated, and yes, I know many of you don't want to hear
it, but he could be brutal. He used to say, "I don't get heart attacks; I
give them."*

*In 1980 when I told him I wanted to be a psychiatrist, he asked me why I didn't want to be a real doctor, why did I want to be a nut doctor and hang out with nuts all day long? It hurt my feelings. He later came to respect what I did and sent me many, many patients. Apparently, he also knew a lot of nuts.*

*Good grief . . . my father is everywhere in my brain . . .*

*From longing for his approval as a child while he was away working to build an empire . . .*
*To adopting his work ethic . . . he was working the day he died, and I suspect I will be working too when my time comes . . .*
*To finally being one of my best friends in the last years of his life and the father who was perfect for me.*

**When grief is prolonged or becomes complicated, get professional help.** In people who are more vulnerable, grief can trigger depressive episodes.

4. **Affirmations to say or meditate on every day:**

   I feel my feelings and cry when needed.
   I choose to heal and move forward.
   I hold on to love and let go of grief.
   The strong person, not the weak one, seeks help when in need.
   Even though I'll never be the same, it is okay to be someone new.

## HOPELESS AND HELPLESS DRAGONS

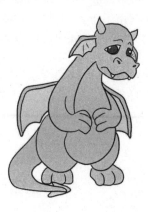

**Origin:** These dragons feed depression, withdrawal, and even suicidal thoughts. People with these dragons have tried to change their circumstances but were unsuccessful, and they have developed what psychologist Martin Seligman calls learned helplessness. They tried and tried and tried, but after a while they learned they were helpless and lost hope. They may have been overwhelmed by stress or conflict and blamed themselves or others because they didn't believe they could change their situation. They have a low sense of self-efficacy. Unfortunately, they carry this negativity forward, and it infects all aspects of their lives. For many people, enduring months of self-isolation due to the coronavirus robbed them of their sense of control over their lives, giving rise to a new generation of Hopeless and Helpless Dragons.

**Triggers:** Any situation that reminds them of feeling overwhelmed or powerless.

**Reactions:** Depression, social withdrawal, resignation, high negativity bias, negative mindset, feelings of hopelessness, helplessness, or powerlessness, blaming self and others, and lack of self-efficacy.

**Movies:** These dragons tend to go for movies that fit their negative mood, such as *Joker, Million Dollar Baby, Schindler's List, What Dreams May Come,* and *The Green Mile.*

**Daniel's Hopeless and Helpless Dragons:** In trying to change my profession of psychiatry by adding neuroimaging and natural ways to heal the brain, I've come up against a decades-long wall of resistance. On the surface, it just makes sense to look at the brains of patients before trying to change them with drugs or other forms of therapy. Making complex diagnoses with no biological information on the organ we treat is just illogical. Initially, I was excited about our work, but the constant stream of criticism, hostility, and dismissiveness from my colleagues almost caused me to lose hope, made me feel anxious and depressed, and forced me to question myself like never before. In 1996, one of my colleagues reported me to the California Medical Board for doing work (brain imaging) outside the standard of care, and they investigated my practice for a year. If I had been found guilty, they could have taken my medical license, which I had worked so hard to obtain. When they concluded the investigation, they found nothing wrong with what I was doing and encouraged me to publish our work, which I've done in many scientific papers. Many times, it felt like I was beating my head against the wall to no avail, leaving me feeling hopeless and helpless. Ultimately, the thousands of positive stories of transformation from our patients and especially from people close to me—such as my nephew Andrew, whose story I told in a six-minute video that has almost 40 million views[36]—helped to rescue me from these dragons.

### Tools to tame your Hopeless and Helpless Dragons

1. **Do you recognize Hopeless and Helpless Dragons in your life?** Are you feeling blue, stuck in a situation, paralyzed to take action, or powerless?

2. **Find the upside:** If you've ever felt hopeless or helpless, you have an easier time understanding others in tough situations. You can develop empathy for people who have felt powerless.

3. **Strategies:**

   **Create a positivity bias.** Purposefully start each day on a positive note. As soon as you awaken or your feet hit the floor in the morning, start the day by saying, "Today is going to be a great day" out loud. Since your mind is prone to negativity, unless you train and discipline it, it will find stress in the upcoming day. When you direct your thoughts to *Today is going to be a great day*, your unconscious brain will help you uncover the reasons why it will be so.

   When I was on a 20-city tour for public television, I woke up in a different city every morning. My brain used to anticipate everything that could go wrong, including the hassles of travel, causing me to feel lousy; but after I learned to start the day with "Today is going to be a great day," I thought of all the wonderful people I'd meet or the lives that might be changed by our work, and I enjoyed the tour very much. We have a choice in where we direct our attention, even in hard times. This simple strategy can make a powerfully positive difference in your life.

Likewise, at the end of the day, write down or meditate on *What went well today?* Doing this will set up your dreams to be more positive, giving you a better night's sleep. Research has also shown that people who did this exercise were happier and less depressed at one-month and six-month follow-ups.[37] This simple exercise has been found to help people in stressful jobs develop more positive emotions.[38] I love doing this because it helps me remember wonderful moments I might have forgotten in my busy life. I even did this the night after my father died, and surprisingly, many things had gone well that day. I received about a thousand loving text messages, my siblings and I all rallied to be there for my mom, and Tana was with me every minute to support me. Ending my day by focusing on these things buoyed my spirits and helped me drift off to sleep.

**Train your brain in gratitude.** Gratitude directs your attention to positive feelings and away from negative ones. Dr. Hans Selye, considered one of the pioneers of stress research, wrote, "Nothing erases unpleasant thoughts more effectively than conscious concentration on pleasant ones."[39] If I could bottle gratitude and appreciation, I would. The benefits far outweigh most of the medications I prescribe, without any side effects. A wealth of research suggests that a daily practice of gratitude, as simple as writing down several things you're grateful for every day, can improve your happiness, mood, self-esteem, resilience, health, looks, productivity, relationships, personality, career, and longevity.

To enhance gratitude, add appreciation, which is gratitude outwardly expressed to build bridges between people. Expressing support and appreciation to others decreases the stress response in the brain much more powerfully than receiving support.[40] To supercharge joyful thinking, get in the daily habit of writing down the name of one person you appreciate and why; then share your feelings with that person with a quick email, text, or call. Try not to repeat anyone in 30 days. This exercise will help you build many bridges of goodwill.

---

*It is better for your brain to give than to receive.*

---

**Write down your accomplishments and strengths.** I once treated a Grammy Award–winning artist who had sold hundreds of millions of records. His brain was only listening to his Hopeless and Helpless Dragons and focused on what was wrong in his life rather than the many things that were right. When I had him write out his accomplishments, he felt much better.

During my first session with Jimmy, the man you read about in the introduction, and his wife, I went to my whiteboard and had them tell me about his strengths. Here's the list: problem solver, persistent, hard worker, loyal, giving, believes in God, humble, organized, servant leader, forgiving, survivor, overcomer, helpful, social, likable, good with people, compassionate, and great father. This helped soothe the Hopeless and Helpless Dragons in his head.

**Get your brain healthy**, especially with strategies that help depression, such as increasing consumption of colorful fruits and vegetables, limiting processed foods, and taking omega-3 fatty acids. Find specific strategies to help heal depression in my book *The End of Mental Illness*.

4. **Affirmations to say or meditate on every day:**

I am worth it.
I can ask for help when I need it.
I have hope for the future.
Today is going to be a great day.
What went well today?

## ANCESTRAL DRAGONS

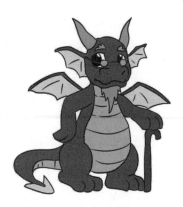

**Origin:** These are your parents' or grandparents' issues passed down to you through their genes, behaviors, or cultural expectations. Their anxieties, fears, prejudices, preconceived notions, political affiliations, and more become yours. For example, children and grandchildren of Holocaust survivors have a higher risk of anxiety disorders and post-traumatic stress disorder (PTSD). In a similar way, 9/11 survivors; Cambodian and Rwanda genocide survivors; those who survived abandonment; people who have had a loved one die by suicide; anyone who has lived in a war zone; or those who have experienced the early death of a child, parent, or sibling often have their nervous system so deeply affected that it changes the nature of their genes to impact their offspring for generations. For example, children of a parent struggling with PTSD are three times more likely to have PTSD themselves. Thirty percent of kids with a parent who served in Iraq or Afghanistan and developed PTSD had similar symptoms. Native American teens on reservations have the highest suicide rate in the Western Hemisphere. In some places it is 10 to 19 times higher than other American teens and young adults.[41] It is as if the massacres against Native Americans continue to this day. Some scholars believe generational grief is fueling the epidemic.

Let's also look at black Americans who have endured racism and mistreatment for about 20 generations. Compared to white adults, they are more likely to have feelings of worthlessness, hopelessness, and sadness. Think of the killing of George Floyd in 2020. It dredged up the Ancestral Dragons for the black community, who felt the hurts not only of this present-day social injustice, but also of all the racial assaults from more than 400 years. The Ancestral Dragons intensified the outrage.

Fear, anxiety, and perhaps even hatred often have ancestral origins. If you are afraid of something and have no idea why, go back through your genealogy to look for any clues that the fear may actually have something to do with your ancestors' experiences. In a large study, children of depressed parents had smaller volume in the pleasure centers of the brain, making the children more vulnerable to depression themselves.[42] And the societal traumas keep coming. A 2020 paper in *JAMA Internal Medicine* suggested that the aftermath of physical distancing and COVID-19 will bring a rise in anxiety, depression, substance abuse, loneliness, and domestic violence.[43] It is likely that global trauma will impact future generations.

Ancestral Dragons might also rear their heads to try to fix a past relationship that was filled with pain. For example, if you grew up in a home with an alcoholic or drug abuser, you might find yourself falling in love with people who struggle with addictions. If you don't work through painful relationships from the past, they can come back to bite you in the present.

**Triggers:** Being the age of a parent or grandparent when they had their trauma. Unknown cultural expectations, or thoughts of what you should do to make your family proud or accepting of you.

**Reactions:** Reluctant compliance, rebellion, feeling guilty or as though you are a disappointment, or anxiety for little to no reason, unexplainable fears.

One of my patients, Jenny, 44, stayed in a destructive marriage 20 years longer than she knew was good for her. The one sticking point was that she could never sleep alone in a house. During therapy, we discovered that her mother grew up in a violent neighborhood in St. Louis and was raped when she was a young woman. Her mother's anxiety pervaded Jenny's upbringing. She was always hesitant to allow Jenny to do sleepovers. One time her mother went through Jenny's friend's whole house before she would let Jenny stay over. Jenny was so embarrassed she never asked to go to another sleepover. Sometimes your anxiety is not yours.

**Movies:** These dragons love historical movies, such as *The King's Speech*, *Braveheart*, *Gandhi*, *Saving Private Ryan*, and *Glory*.

**Daniel's Ancestral Dragons:** In looking at my family history, I inherited many traits, fears, and unconscious beliefs from my immigrant great-grandparents and grandparents who were risk takers, merchants, and unaccepting of the status quo. They escaped the repression of the Ottoman Empire and the great famine during World War I, seeking a better life. The mindset of both my parents also influences me; they grew up during the Great Depression and World War II with issues around family, security, hard work, and money.

Being of Lebanese descent, Middle Eastern issues were always front and center in our home and passionately discussed. My grandfather had owned a home in Haifa, Palestine, which was taken from him when Israel became an independent country in 1948.

In 1976, I was on the speech team in college and won the California State Championship for Peace Oratory, arguing for a two-state solution in the Middle East. I won nearly all of the speech competitions I entered that year except one at Pasadena City College, where I came in last out of 10 speakers. On the comment card one of the judges wrote, "That is such a big solution from such a little man." The comment fired up my Inferior, Angry, Judgmental, and Ancestral Dragons. I wonder how many dragons from the past haunt the issues of the Middle East, making peace so hard to achieve.

I also have significant ancestral trauma. When my paternal grandfather was a young man, his younger brother was killed in a train accident while driving a car. So my grandfather never drove a car. My paternal grandmother's father was murdered by bandits in Mexico while working on bringing the family to the United States. After that happened, her mother could not take care of her and her sister, so they were sent to live in an orphanage in Bethlehem. The death of her father and separation from her mother deeply affected her. Perhaps some of my childhood anxiety was not all mine.

### Tools to tame your Ancestral Dragons

1. **Do you recognize Ancestral Dragons in your life?** Do you have seemingly unfounded fears or anxieties? This may be a sign that these feelings come from a past generation.

2. **Find the upside:** We all inherit positive and negative traits and experiences from our parents, grandparents, and other ancestors. Focus on the benefits and good characteristics that you gained from your family of origin.

3. **Strategies:**

   **Know your family history in as much detail as you can.** Talk to your parents, grandparents, and whoever is the family historian. It can help you understand some of your automatic reactions that seemed puzzling to you before. Close your eyes and visualize your family members (mother, father, grandparents, and so on) and see if you can feel what they were feeling, to see if it at all relates to your own struggles.

**Work to separate your ancestors' issues from your own issues so that you can live in the present rather than the past.** This may require professional help. If you sense Ancestral Dragons breathing fire on your emotional brain, read *It Didn't Start with You* by Mark Wolynn.

**Reduce exposure to triggers.** This doesn't mean avoiding your family's past or pretending it didn't exist. Rather, it means you don't have to subject yourself to painful reminders that cause you to relive the trauma over and over.

**Design a new future.** Focus on creating a future for yourself that is no longer stuck in the pain of ancestral trauma. Imagine yourself living in a way that you are not weighed down by the chains of your ancestors. When you can envision this, you may break the cycle of ancestral trauma.

**Try somatic experiencing,** a type of trauma therapy that involves paying close attention to your inner body sensations as a way to regulate emotions. It is similar to mindfulness practices that help you tune in to your body to achieve a desired emotional state. A professional can guide you through the process more effectively.

4. **Affirmations to say or meditate on every day:**

I appreciate and honor my ancestors.
Sometimes my anxiety may not be from my lifetime but another lifetime.
I work to live in the present and the future.

## ARE DRAGONS FROM THE PAST TERRORIZING YOUR BUSINESS?

What gives dragons fuel for the flames? When we get our feelings hurt, when we feel invisible, inadequate, angry, or ashamed, our amygdala activates, and we feel anxious, irritated, and out of sorts. Our amygdala is constantly scanning the world to protect us from danger. If we see trouble about to happen, such as a small child near the top of a staircase, our amygdala might sound the alarm, causing us to jump up and protect the child before something bad happens. The purpose of the amygdala is to scan for danger, alert us as soon as it senses it, and then help us get ready to react to it—whatever we might perceive the danger to be. But is the danger in the present or the past?

The crazy part is that your amygdala doesn't know the difference between a child in danger and a critical comment made by a coworker. Your amygdala, especially if it has been sensitized by hurts in the past, is constantly looking for trouble, listening to your coworker's tone of voice, words, actions, as well as what you think his or her intentions may be. If your coworker triggers one of your dragons, you are more likely to overreact to the situation, which in turn may trigger their dragons, causing an unnecessary war.

At the end of an all-day planning meeting with her team, Carrie, a chief executive officer, wrapped up the day with a long sigh and asked if anyone else had anything to say. Mike, the company's chief financial officer, wanted to express his concerns about the spending in the marketing department, but he felt hesitant because he hated conflict (Anxious Dragons) and sensed the marketing director, Christian, might get angry with him (Angry Dragons). Yet he knew if he didn't say anything, Carrie might think he was shirking his responsibilities (Responsibility Dragons), so he spoke up. Almost immediately, Christian could feel his stomach tighten and his face redden, and he lashed out, calling Mike a jerk and telling the whole executive team they didn't understand how hard his job was. Taken aback, Carrie tried to calm things down, but the outburst left the team feeling stressed out and deflated the whole next week, until she could get Mike and Christian in her office to work things out.

What happened?

The way you know your amygdala is being activated is when you feel afraid, angry, or stressed. Your body tells you with a racing heart, sweaty palms, chest tightness, or trouble breathing. Don't allow your Dragons from the Past to ruin your business.

## BE AWARE THAT DRAGONS FROM THE PAST TEND TO RESURFACE WHEN YOU HAVE CHILDREN

Dragons can be quiet for many years, even decades, and then come roaring back to burn you when you have children. That's what happened to Prince William, the Duke of Cambridge. In a BBC documentary, he revealed that fatherhood unexpectedly dredged up painful emotions he had experienced after the death of his mother, Diana, Princess of Wales. In the interview about parenthood, he says, "When you've been through something traumatic in life . . . my mother dying when I was younger, your emotions come back in leaps and bounds. . . . Things come out of the blue that you don't ever expect or that maybe you think you've dealt with."[44] Becoming a parent can trigger the Death Dragons, Grief and Loss Dragons, Wounded Dragons, and many others. People often unconsciously relive their own pasts as their children grow. Whenever children are a certain age, parents tend to remember the traumas and joys when they were that age. For example, when their children go to kindergarten, they remember what kindergarten was like for them. If that was a time of separation anxiety or being bullied, creating your Anxious or Angry Dragons, you are more vulnerable to those feelings and have no idea why you are anxious or irritable.

When Stephanie, a marketing executive in a happy marriage and mother of an eight-year-old daughter, started having panic attacks that seemed to come out of the blue, her family doctor prescribed Xanax, an anti-anxiety medication. She was uncomfortable taking it and came to an Amen Clinic. When I had her close her eyes, go back to the last panic attack she had, and tell me what she was thinking and feeling, she told me, "Frightened and had to get away from something but didn't know what." I then asked her to go back in her mind to the very first time she felt that way. In about 20 seconds, she started to cry and said that when she was eight years old at her first sleepover, her friend's father fondled her. She had completely repressed the memory. Her daughter's request to go to her first sleepover triggered Stephanie's Wounded Dragons and caused a fight between Stephanie and her husband. Knowing what had happened allowed us to work through the trauma.

## YOU CAN REWRITE YOUR DRAGON STORIES

The good news is that Dragons from the Past do not have to control you. Begin to rewrite their stories. Remember when Jimmy, from the introduction, had to give an impact statement at 12 years old during the penalty phase of his father's murder trial? The thought he internalized was *If I fail, I could kill my father,* which triggered his fear of public speaking and his lifelong Anxious Dragons. Together we rewrote his story: "I am strong and helped to save my father from the death penalty. I am powerful and brave." He needed to go back in his mind and love his 12-year-old self, rather than allow the 12-year-old's anxiety to continue to control him. He could soothe his inner child as a good parent would. He began to see his life through the lens of post-traumatic growth, rather than through trauma and being a victim.

How can you start to rewrite the stories you've been playing in your head? Here are five simple steps.

1. Identify the dragons blocking your path to success and work to retrain them by looking at their triggers and upsides.

2. See yourself as the creator of your story: past, present, and future. I used to tell myself that my father never spent any time with us. For decades, I remembered him with bitterness and believed I was justified for having those negative feelings. Then when I was 50, he gave all his kids copies of home movies he took when we were young. It had many moments with him at the park, pool, or parties playing with us. My Insignificant and Angry Dragons had been lying to me, which had a negative impact on our relationship. Being able to rewrite the story from a more accurate, mature standpoint dramatically helped our relationship and how I felt inside.

3. Know what you want. Write it down and ask yourself, *What can I do today to start getting what I want?* You don't have to do everything today, just one small thing. I often tell my patients who feel frozen by fear that they don't have to react all at once, just move their pinky finger to signal they can do something.

4. Remember that where you focus your attention always determines how you feel. If I focused on my critics, I would feel criticized, angry, small, and like a victim. But if I focus on all the people we've helped, I feel happy and purposeful. I have a choice on the arc and ending of the story.

5. Realize it is never too late to change your story. Start today. As the title character in the film *The Curious Case of Benjamin Button* said, "It's never too late . . . to be whoever you wanna be. . . . You can change or stay the same. There are no rules to this thing. . . . I hope you live a life you're proud of, and if you find that you're not, I hope you have the strength to start all over again."[45]

# QUIET THE THEY, THEM, AND OTHER DRAGONS

## DON'T LET THEIR DRAGONS PICK FIGHTS WITH YOURS

*I learned long ago never wrestle with a pig, you both get dirty and only the pig likes it.*
**UNKNOWN**

*What you think of me is none of my business.*
**TERRY COLE-WHITTAKER**

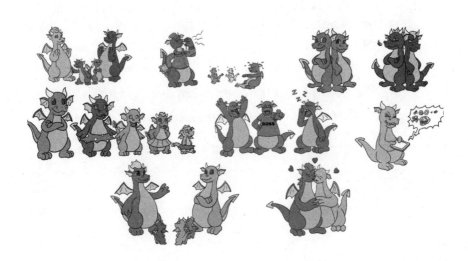

In addition to the Dragons from the Past, which breathe fire on your emotional brain, your mind is always listening to the words and actions of other people (They, Them, and Other Dragons), both alive and dead, who each have their own Dragons from the Past. That's why relationships are often messy. Unless you are careful, you are never just dealing with the moment; you are also dealing with all the moments of all the people involved, which is why heeding Byron Katie's words can be so healing: "It's not your job to like me. It's mine."[1]

In times of stress, such as when families, couples, and roommates were cooped up for months to try to slow the spread of COVID-19, there was no escape from the They, Them, and Other Dragons. Being in close quarters escalated the fire breathing among these beasts. We were also all subjected to conflicting societal messages that left us feeling confused, sad, anxious, frustrated, angry, and fearful, and those fueled our own Dragons from the Past.

Let's start by asking who "they" are. Growing up, my mother said (and maybe yours did too), "If you don't have something good to say, don't say anything at all. 'They' wouldn't like it." I often wondered who "they" were. Have you noticed people say things like "They said this . . ." "They said that . . ." "They think you should dress better, be taller, smarter, stronger, or more talented." "They" are the collective voices in our heads that are constantly judging or criticizing our thoughts, actions, words, and the way we look. Let's briefly explore nine of the They, Them, and Other Dragons that may be unconsciously impacting your happiness, relationships, and success.

---

*Be kind to everyone you meet, because we
are all fighting our own dragons.*

**ANONYMOUS**

---

# PARENT DRAGONS

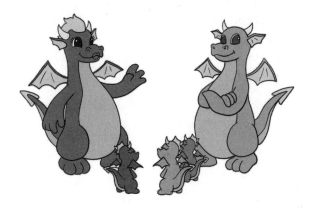

Your brain is always listening to the voices of your mother or father (or mother or father figures) criticizing you or pushing you to be better. Most of us heard their words so often they became ingrained into the nerve tracks in our brain. Have you ever found yourself repeating to your own children the words your parents told you, even though you promised yourself you never would? Our brains are always listening to the words of our parents—their guidance, expectations, approval or disapproval, and much more. When stay-at-home orders were put in place during the pandemic, you may have heard your Parent Dragons telling you to follow the rules and get prepared.

Jimmy's gang leader father often said he did hard things to "test his mettle," to see how tough he was. In prison, he told Jimmy he would purposefully go into a cell with a gang member who he suspected might want to kill him, just to see if he could survive the attack. Knowing this about his father led Jimmy to work hard at things he found challenging, even when they were not the best fit for him.

I used to think persistence was a virtue until I realized stalkers are also persistent. I never want my children or grandchildren to give up too easily when things are hard, but I also do not want them frustrated by sticking with things that are not a good fit or possible for them. If I had wanted to be the center for the Los Angeles Lakers basketball team, no matter how much I tried, it still would have never happened.

If your mother was amazing, thank her often. Children from homes where the father was an alcoholic suffered, but when the mother was an alcoholic, it was much more stressful for the kids. Why? In virtually every society, mothers are the primary caretakers for children. When she is impaired or absent, it has a much more negative effect on children.

**When the Parent Dragons are triggered,** you feel like you've done something wrong, you are not good enough or supported, and you are motivated to work harder.

**What do you need to listen to or leave behind?** Focus on the positive parental messaging you received, and flip the rest around to use it to prove them wrong.

## SIBLING AND BIRTH ORDER DRAGONS

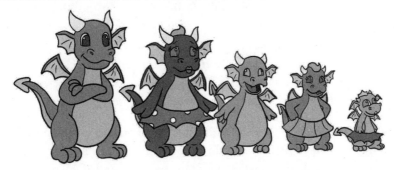

Your brain is always listening to your birth order and the voices of your siblings, who were often competing with you for your parents' attention. One of the reasons the holidays may be hard for people is that their siblings continually bring up embarrassing stories from childhood. Since they have known you longer than anyone else, none of your past weird behaviors are ever left behind. Last Christmas I found myself irritated with my older sister who brought up, for what seemed like the fiftieth time, how I lit the couch on fire when I was five years old. Thankfully, my younger sister, who was four at the time and my accomplice with the matches that day, spoke up and told everyone, also for the fiftieth time, how she hid behind me in the closet, while I protected her and took the spanking for us both. Depending on whose perspective you hear, I am either a pyromaniac or a loyal friend.

Your brain is also listening to your place in your family. Although the research is mixed and there is immense individual variation, birth order certainly may impact development.[2]

**Firstborn children** (firstborn, first child born of a specific gender, a child whose next-closest sibling is five or more years older) get 3,000 more hours of attention from their parents, so they tend to walk earlier, talk earlier, and have higher IQ scores. Typically, in larger families (family size matters), oldest kids have more responsibility at home (babysitting and chores), which can increase their sense of confidence and responsibility. They start at higher-paying jobs,[3] although their younger siblings tend to catch up. Firstborns often fill positions of authority, including 14 of 45 US Presidents (only seven were youngest children) and 21 of the first 23 NASA astronauts who went to space, but are more likely to have narcissistic traits[4] and be the worst drivers.[5]

**Middle children** (yours truly) have the fewest pictures in the family photo albums, tend to be mediators (like psychiatrists) and loyal. They generally are open to compromise, often at their own expense, and avoid conflict (they get beaten up by the older ones). Because they often are unspoiled, they tend to be less frustrated by the demands of life (I lived in the Mojave Desert for two years and was perfectly happy). They tend to have fewer emotional problems and are less likely to be diagnosed with ADHD[6] but are more likely to be mavericks (my father and I were both middle kids) and push against authority. They leave home earlier. The apparent "disadvantages" of middle children may help them be more empathetic and independent.

**Youngest children** tend to be charming and social but can also blame others. When my next-to-youngest was little, she blamed her older brother for everything that went bad. Her nickname for him was Didi, and "Didi did it." One day when she spilled her milk, she said, "Didi did it." When her mother said Didi wasn't home because he spent the night at a friend's house, she said, "Didi came home, spilled the milk, and then left."[7] Youngest children view their older siblings as bigger, faster, and smarter, and they may attempt to differentiate themselves by being more rebellious. Since they had the fewest limits, they are more likely to take risks. If both spouses are two youngest children, they are more likely to get into debt. Latter-born children have a higher incidence of drug and alcohol treatment.[8]

**Only children** are similar to both firstborn and youngest children, and they are more ambitious than any other group if they are from middle-class families.[9] They are more likely to be academically successful, happy, flexible in their thinking, and creative, but they also are perceived by others to be more self-centered.[10] Another downside is that in numerous studies, only children have a higher incidence of obesity. If they're spoiled, they have another set of dragons to deal with (more on that in a moment).

We tend to spend more time with those who are like us. "Firstborns are more likely to associate with firstborns, middle-borns with middle-borns, last-borns with last-borns, and only children with only children."[11]

**When the Sibling and Birth Order Dragons are triggered,** you may feel a sense of responsibility toward others (firstborn), rebel against authority (middle child), use charm to get your way (youngest child), or think first about yourself (only child).

**What do you need to listen to or leave behind?** Take responsibility for your own life, but don't do too much for others (oldest child). Innovate but don't denigrate others in the process (middle child). Back up your charm with smarts and hard work (youngest child), and work to be inclusive and think more about others (only child).

# CHILDREN DRAGONS

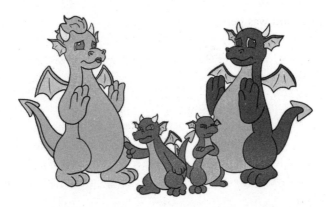

Your brain is always listening to the voices of your children who often (although not always) adore you through their elementary school years then push away and criticize you during their adolescent and young adult years. As much as it hurts for parents who experience this rejection, it is normal and part of processes called individuation and identity formation. Knowing that helps to soften the injury to our egos. When my kids would tell me I was crazy, I'd respond, "Insanity is hereditary; you get it from your children."

At 41, one of my patients, Melissa, who had struggled for years to get pregnant was ecstatic when she finally gave birth to twin daughters. Being a mother was the greatest joy of her life, and she was determined to be the loving and caring parent she never had. Her own mother had been neglectful, leaving Melissa with Invisible Dragons. Melissa devoted herself and enjoyed a strong relationship with her daughters until they hit age 12. That's when the loving bond they shared seemed to disintegrate, and her daughters started alternating between ignoring Melissa and saying hurtful things to her. Melissa felt her Invisible Dragons return with a vengeance. That's when she came to see me. I helped her understand that the rejection she was feeling was a normal part of the maturation process, and I helped her work on taming her Dragons from the Past. Melissa learned to let her daughters develop their own identities, and in time, the girls stopped pulling away and started seeking their mom's advice and her company.

Since you will hear your children's approval or disapproval for the rest of your life, once you have them, work on building a great relationship with them. You do not do this by spoiling them. You do it with actual physical time, active listening, and being firm and kind with them. Some of my favorite books on raising healthy children include my book, *New Skills for Frazzled*

*Parents, Parenting with Love and Logic* by Foster W. Cline and Jim Fay, and *The Entitlement Cure* by John Townsend.

**When the Children Dragons are triggered,** you feel hurt, ignored, and insignificant—or you can feel connected, confident, protective, and proud.

**What do you need to listen to or leave behind?** When you hear or remember the stinging comments from your teenagers, pair them with the loving words you heard when they were younger or after they reached adulthood; this will keep your emotions balanced. When you don't hear from them, remind yourself that you have raised healthy, independent adults, and the fact that they don't need you for every decision they make means you've done a good parenting job.

## TEACHER AND COACH DRAGONS

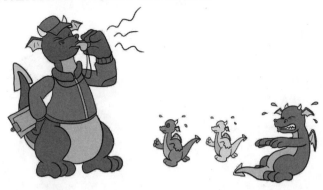

Your brain is always listening to the voices of your teachers, who graded your intelligence and effort, and your coaches, who noticed your abilities and flaws. The quality of these people is so important, as you hear their voices for decades after they have left your life. Here are two diametrically opposed examples.

In my second year of college, I decided that I wanted to go to medical school. At the time, I was on the speech team and competed in persuasive oratory. When I told our coach about my plans to go to medical school, she told me her younger brother didn't get into medical school after several tries and he was twice as smart as I was. In other words, she told me I didn't have a chance. When I told my dad what she said, he told me not to spend much time around her, as people are contagious.

Later, when I was a second-year medical student, I had a pathology professor who was incredibly gifted and kind. He was funny and interesting, and he made his class presentations pertinent and practical. Even better, he was famous for making dead facts come alive. He made a tough subject enjoyable. He also nurtured positive relationships with the students. I remember piling into his car with three other classmates to go to a funeral home in Henryetta, Oklahoma, to perform our first autopsy. He was the master pathologist, and by cultivating a close relationship with him, we learned more than the dead facts. We began to understand the workings of a superb pathologist's mind in solving medical problems. He cemented my interest in medicine.

How have your teachers and coaches influenced you?

**When the Teacher and Coach Dragons are triggered,** you feel stupid, unqualified, and incapable of learning—or you feel empowered to live up to your potential.

**What do you need to listen to or leave behind?** Listen to their encouraging words and constructive critiques. Leave behind their harsh criticisms or bad behaviors.

# FRIENDS, POPULAR KIDS, BULLIES, AND MEAN GIRLS DRAGONS

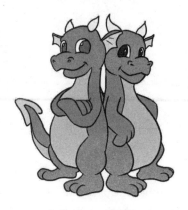 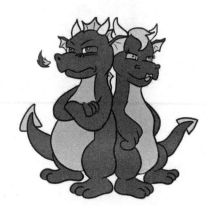

Your brain is always listening to the voices of your past friends, as well as the popular kids, bullies, and mean girls from when you were growing up. These relationships soothe your dragons (good friends) or cause them to breathe fire (bullies and mean girls). Humans are a relational species, and formative relationships have a lasting effect. To the chagrin of parents, peer relationships often have more sway on development during adolescence than parent-teen relationships.

Go back in your mind to assess the impact your early relationships had on your dragons, and reevaluate them through the lens of knowing that each of these people had their own dragons too. For example, the popular kids who ignored you may have been ignored by their parents who worked all the time, the bullies may have been raised by a bully at home, and the mean girls may have been dealing with an angry alcoholic father. Taking time to reflect on these relationships from a broader perspective often helps to dial down the heat they blow on your emotional brain areas.

My three best friends during adolescence all lived in stressful home environments. Two had mothers who were alcoholics; the other had a violent alcoholic father. Their moods could be up and down, and I would often personalize it. One offered me marijuana for the first time and then asked out my girlfriend. I ended the relationship with my friend but became sensitive to betrayal and had more issues with trust. Looking back with the understanding of an adult and my psychiatric training helped to soothe my inner Friends Dragons.

Your brain is also listening to your current friends and relationships. When you confide in them, know they are not just giving you simple advice. Their own dragons are influencing what they tell you.

**When Friends, Popular Kids, Bullies, and Mean Girl Dragons are triggered**, you feel confident, likable, and supported—or you feel betrayed, unworthy of being liked, and lonely.

**What do you need to listen to or leave behind?** Listen to the friendly and encouraging sentiments of your pals, and remember that the unkind words from bullies and mean girls were likely a reflection of their own insecurities.

# FORMER, CURRENT, AND PROSPECTIVE LOVER DRAGONS

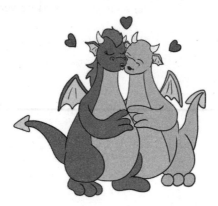

Your brain is always listening to the group of Former, Current, and Prospective Lover Dragons. These are the most emotionally charged dragons of all, which is why they can make you more upset than any of the other ones, especially when the relationship goes sour. Your brain is always listening to the criticisms and encouragements of past sweethearts, the words and deeds of your current spouse, and even the imagined attitudes and judgment of future relationships. Never forget that all of these past, present, and future people have their own dragons.

Your brain is always listening to love. Love is a drug primarily housed in your brain, not your heart. When you say, "I love you with all my heart," it's more accurate to say, "I love you with all my brain," but it doesn't sound nearly as romantic. When you say, "You broke my heart," it really means your brain is in pain, which can cause chest pain, but it is not primarily cardiac in origin. *Sweetheart, my heart, heart* are terms of endearment, but shouldn't they be *sweetbrain, my brain, brain*? Maybe.

Anthropologist Helen Fisher published a study using brain scans of college students who viewed pictures of someone special along with those of acquaintances.[12] The pictures of their loved ones activated the pleasure centers in the brain, rich in the "feel good" neurotransmitter dopamine that's involved with attention and the motivation to pursue and acquire rewards. That is why, when you do find a match on a dating site or at work or church, the high of new love can feel like an addiction with its euphoria, craving, withdrawal, and the need for more and more to feel good.[13] New love works in the same areas of the brain as cocaine and can cause people to feel giddy, anxious, uncertain, obsessed; irrationally notice the positive and completely miss the negative; make poor decisions; have trouble sleeping; and feel as if they are on a roller coaster. When the high of new love wears off, the other person's faults are easy to see, and couples can more rationally decide to stay together or to separate. For this reason you should be very cautious about marrying someone within the first few months of meeting. You can't be certain if your brain is listening to the actual person or a drug-induced illusion.

Lasting love, even after 20 years or more, can still activate the brain's pleasure centers but in different ways from new love. Lasting love provides a deeper sense of bonding and connection, peace, happiness, and warmth—more akin to the warmth of heroin than the jolt of cocaine. The feeling of being high on heroin was once anonymously described as "being cradled to sleep by God, wrapped up in a warm, luxurious blanket that shields you from all your worldly fears, angers, and pains." While the pain of a new love breakup feels awful, leaving a long-term love relationship is typically much worse. Many people describe it as feeling as if their skin is being ripped off while they are awake. It is often associated with symptoms similar to heroin withdrawal—diarrhea, nausea, depression, and a sense of hopelessness that can go on for months, together with anxiety, panic, and sleeplessness.

For many, love has turned into a video game. Amen Clinics collaborated with *The Dr. Oz Show* and did a brain imaging–Tinder experiment with several 30-somethings to determine the effect of the dating app on mood and focus. If they were lucky enough to get a "swipe right" (meaning their pictures and short bio were liked), it increased activity in the pleasure and mood centers of their brains; if, however, there were fewer "swipes right" and more "swipes left" (indicating rejection), their brains were more vulnerable to pain and depression.

**When Former, Current, and Prospective Lover Dragons are triggered**, you feel loved, confident, and sexy—or you feel abandoned, betrayed, unlovable, and hurt. You may find it hard to trust potential new lovers, or you may push them away without understanding why.

**What do you need to listen to or leave behind?** Reframe any harsh words from former lovers so you can learn from the mistakes you've made in past relationships without beating yourself up.

## INTERNET TROLL DRAGONS

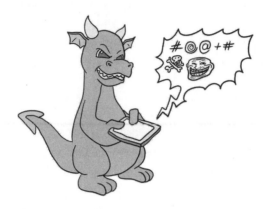

Your brain is always listening to the voices of the people or bots on social media and the internet trolls who criticize you for sport. Unfortunately, this is happening at younger and younger ages. I have a nine-year-old niece who was bullied by an ex-friend on social media. Many of my teenage patients have taken or allowed others to take inappropriate pictures of them they thought were being shared privately. When those images ended up on the internet, my patients experienced intense embarrassment, shame, and often suicidal thoughts or behavior.

A number of celebrity patients constantly check the internet to see what other people write about them. It often becomes an addiction and hijacks their brains. Miley Cyrus used to be one of them. While going cold turkey has helped many of them regain their sense of emotional balance, Miley took a slightly different approach. On her Instagram Live show called *Bright Minded*, she talked about how the *B* in *Bright Minds* is for the Blessings/ Curses of social media. I helped her understand how to minimize its curses by limiting her exposure to internet trolls. Rather than going cold turkey, she stays focused on the blessings of social media, which is the ability to connect with her fans in a positive and meaningful way.

On the internet people are often anonymous and write whatever unfil-tered, mean, hurtful thought comes into their brains. Of course, there are many pluses to technology, but they do not come without a steep price for many people.

If your business is online, then your business has to manage the com-ments. If you are the one being attacked—as I have been brutally attacked over the years by colleagues—have someone else from your team manage your sites; it will help keep the Internet Troll Dragons at bay and out of your head.

**When the Internet Troll Dragons are triggered**, you believe every hateful word you read online, making you feel worthless, helpless, and untalented.

**What do you need to listen to or leave behind?** If possible, avoid reading comments so you don't give the internet trolls a voice. Remind yourself that if people are taking the time to write something about you online, even if it's negative, at least it means you're doing something that's making an impact.

# OTHER PEOPLE'S DRAGONS ARE CONTAGIOUS

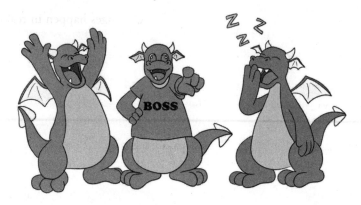

Your brain is always listening to the voices of many other dragons, including bosses, coworkers, religious leaders, politicians, store clerks, news reporters, and media personalities. We'll look at those in depth in section 5. These dragons can be critical, hurtful, attacking, competing, and indifferent; or they can be encouraging, positive, comforting, and engaged. If you watch some news channels, the political leaders are the personification of the devil; if you watch other channels, they are saints, and you are a fool to think otherwise. If you look at magazines that highlight pretty, skinny models, you will think that is beautiful; if you look at other magazines, you will think a different look is most attractive. Where you bring your attention determines how you feel. As my wife likes to say to her single friends who tell her they meet only difficult men, "It's not all men. It's the ones you choose to give your number to."

Everyone has energy that impacts the brains around them. Intuitively we know that negative people infect a group with stress, while positive people tend to increase everyone's joy. But is there science to back that up? Over the years at Amen Clinics, we've done before-and-after brain imaging studies for a wide variety of interventions from medications, nutritional supplements, hyperbaric oxygen, meditation, hypnosis, and prayer.

One of the more fascinating studies we did was on qi gong (a centuries-old healing practice using targeted coordination movements, breathing, and meditation), where a qi gong master directed healing energy to five people. We performed before-and-after SPECT scans and QEEG scans, which measure electrical activity in the brain. The SPECT scans showed increased blood flow in four of the five subjects. The QEEG scans showed immediate changes in all of the subjects; I remember how amazed our neurology expert was when he was seeing the changes happen in real time on the computer screen.

We are often manipulated by television, radio, streaming services, social media, internet ads, magazines, shopping malls, and watercooler discussions at work. Be mindful of the noise you allow in your head.

# TAME THE THOUGHTS THAT FUEL YOUR DRAGONS

## HOW CHALLENGING 100 OF YOUR WORST THOUGHTS CAN HEAL YOUR LIFE

*A thought is harmless unless we believe it. It's not our thoughts, but the attachment to our thoughts, that causes suffering. Attaching to a thought means believing that it's true, without inquiring. A belief is a thought that we've been attaching to, often for years.*

**BYRON KATIE,** *LOVING WHAT IS: FOUR QUESTIONS THAT CAN CHANGE YOUR LIFE*

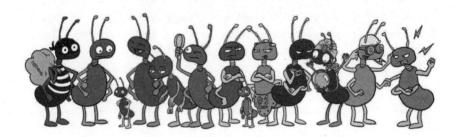

**W**hen I was a young psychiatrist, I used a technique called biofeedback to help understand and treat my patients. Biofeedback uses instruments to measure hand temperature, sweat gland activity, muscle tension, breathing rate, heart rate, and brain wave patterns. If we know how your body reacts to stress, we can teach you to soothe it. Your conscious and unconscious brain expresses its aspirations, worries, fears, stress, love, joy, hatred, and happiness through your body's reactions. Knowing this, I developed a word association test to see how my patients' bodies respond to certain words and concepts. I hook them up to biofeedback equipment as I would to a lie detector machine and then ask them to think about certain words. Some of the words are innocuous, such as *telephone*, *book*, or *paper clip*, and other words have more emotional meanings, such as *mother*, *father*, *siblings*, *job*, *children*, and *spouse*.

Most people have only small physiological reactions to innocuous words but much larger reactions to emotionally loaded words. For example, if I say *baseball* or *train*, there is usually little movement in the biofeedback equipment, unless a person loves a baseball team or collects model trains. However, when I say words like *mother* or *father*, I usually see a significant change. If *mother* is a positive concept in the person's life, like mine is for me, the changes move in a positive direction: heart and breathing rates slow, muscles become more relaxed, hands become warmer and drier. If *mother* is associated with painful or stressful memories, the change usually goes in a stressful direction: heart and breathing rates escalate, muscles become tense, hands become colder, and sweat gland activity increases.

Through biofeedback, I've learned that your brain is always listening and responding to every thought you have, especially the stressful and positive ones. The thousands of thoughts you have every day are based on myriad factors, including the Dragons from the Past; They, Them, Other Dragons; genetics; past experiences; sensory input; dreams; what you had for dinner last night; and the health of your gut bacteria. Negative thoughts cause your brain to immediately release chemicals that affect every cell in your body, making you feel bad; while the opposite is also true—positive, happy, hopeful thoughts release chemicals that make you feel good. Your thought patterns can also have long-term effects. Repetitive negative thinking may promote the buildup of the harmful deposits seen in the brains of people with Alzheimer's disease and may increase the risk of dementia, according to a 2020 brain imaging study in *Alzheimer's & Dementia*.[1]

Thoughts are also automatic. They just happen.

*Just because you have a thought has nothing to do with whether it is true.* Thoughts lie. They lie a lot, and it is your uninvestigated or unquestioned thoughts that steal your happiness. If you do not question or correct your erroneous thoughts, you believe them, and you act as if they are 100 percent true. For example, if my Inferior Dragons triggered the thought, *My wife never listens to me*, it would make me feel sad and lonely, and it would fuel my Angry Dragons. If I never questioned the negative thought, even though it isn't true, I would act as if it were true and give myself permission to be irritable with her, making it less likely she would ever *want* to listen to me. Allowing yourself to believe every thought you have is the prescription for anxiety disorders, depression, relationship problems, and chronic illness. You must protect yourself from the thoughts that dragons are speaking to try to steal your happiness.

This became evident when the spread of the coronavirus led to a rampant rise in unhealthy thinking patterns. As I said in several of my Facebook Live chats, in a pandemic, mental hygiene is just as important as washing your hands. We need to disinfect our thoughts. Let me show you how.

---

*Just because you have a thought has nothing to do with whether it is true.*

---

## THE ANTS THAT FUEL YOUR DRAGONS

In the early nineties, I coined the term *automatic negative thoughts* to describe how negativity can infest your brain.[2] Since then, I've written about ANTs in many of my books because they are one of the biggest influences on brain health. The idea came to me after a hard day at work where I had seen four suicidal patients, two teenagers who ran away from home, and two couples who hated their spouses. When I got home that night, there was an ant infestation in my kitchen, where thousands of these insects were trying to take over. As I cleaned them up, the idea came to me that my patients were also infested with ANTs (automatic negative thoughts) that were driving their feelings of depression, hopelessness, helplessness, and irritability.

I knew that if I could teach my patients to eliminate the ANTs, it would also help tame their dragons, and they would feel happier, less anxious, and be better able to get along with others. The next day, I brought a can of ant spray to work and started to teach my patients how to kill the ANTs. Over time, I replaced the ant spray with ant and anteater puppets, which I still use to this day. Early on I saw an eight-year-old boy who had a dog phobia

(Anxious Dragons). Three weeks after I taught him to kill the ANTs, he told me it was an ANT ghost town in his head.[3]

My ANT killing process is based on the work of two mentors: psychiatrist Aaron Beck, who pioneered a school of psychotherapy called cognitive behavior therapy (CBT), which is an effective treatment for anxiety disorders, depression, relationship problems, and even obesity; and Byron Katie, a teacher and author who developed the questions we'll discuss to kill ANTs.

How you feel is often related to the quality of your thoughts. If they are mostly negative, you will feel mostly negative; if they are mostly positive, you will feel mostly positive. ANTs link, stack, and multiply with other ANTs to attack you. For instance, the ANTs grow stronger and increase in number before bed, when you get less sleep, when your blood sugar is low, in winter, right before a woman's menstrual cycle, when you're under stress, and when you lose someone you love. The coronavirus pandemic has led to an ANT infestation unlike anything we've seen before. These ANTs feed your Dragons from the Past, making them stronger and more likely to torture you.

Eliminate the ANTs to help tame dragons and be better able to cope with whatever stresses come your way.

Let me be very clear, I'm not a fan of positive thinking. Positive thinking says you can have the third piece of cheesecake and it won't hurt you. I'm a fan of accurate thinking. I always want you to tell yourself the truth. Accurate thinking leads to better mental health, fewer bad habits, and a happier life, while unbridled positive thinking does not.

As you learn to eliminate the ANTs, your brain will become more disciplined to constantly seek the truth. I'll describe the nine most common ANTs that provide the fuel for emotional suffering and relationship problems, along with which dragons they tend to fuel.

## ANT TYPES

1. All-or-Nothing ANTs: Thinking that things are either all good or all bad

2. Less-Than ANTs: Comparing and seeing yourself as less than others

3. Just-the-Bad ANTs: Seeing only the bad in a situation

4. Guilt-Beating ANTs: Thinking in words like *should, must, ought,* or *have to*

5. Labeling ANTs: Attaching a negative label to yourself or someone else

6. Fortune-Telling ANTs: Predicting the worst possible outcome for a situation with little or no evidence for it

7. Mind-Reading ANTs: Believing you know what other people are thinking even though they haven't told you

8. If-Only and I'll-Be-Happy-When ANTs: Arguing with the past and longing for the future

9. Blaming ANTs: Blaming someone else for your problems

## ALL-OR-NOTHING ANTS *(fuel Judgmental Dragons)*

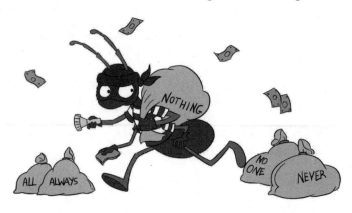

These sneaky ANTs attack whenever you think things are all good or all bad. They don't use words like *sometimes* or *maybe*. These ANTs think in absolute words that make situations *all good* or *all bad*. This is also called black-or-white thinking because it splits reality into light and dark, or good and bad, without acknowledging life's complexities, ambiguities, and nuances. You know these ANTs are around whenever you think in words like *all, always, any, never, no one, nothing, everyone, every time*. These ANTs attack when you believe things are completely right or totally wrong, that people are either friends or enemies, that a day is perfect or terrible, or that you are a total success or a complete failure. These ANTs tell you that it is now or never, that everything that is not good is bad, that you are beautiful or ugly, that you love or hate someone, and so on.

I once saw the runner-up to the television show *The Biggest Loser*. He had lost over 100 pounds. Yet he was depressed because he saw himself as a complete failure since he did not finish first. He beat out many other contestants and literally lost the weight equivalent to a small adult.

All-or-Nothing ANTs make clear, rigid, and lasting distinctions often based on half-truths or lies. They reduce complex concepts into two opposing categories: good or bad. On the surface, these ANTs make you feel better about yourself because you can put people and actions into simple categories. Just open any political news feed and you'll see pundits putting the other side into the all-bad category.

It's easy to spot all-or-nothing thinkers as they tend to see only one side of a situation, ignore evidence to the contrary, and get into heated arguments with people who do not share their views. Yet this stinking thinking pattern obscures judgment, leads to bad decisions, decreases one's ability to understand the world, ruins relationships, and reduces the number of ways to solve problems. No wonder these ANTs fuel Judgmental Dragons.

Here's an example: At Amen Clinics we did the first and largest study on active and retired NFL players. More than half of our retired players were obese, which, as we will see, is very bad for the brain, so we ran a weight-loss group for athletes. One obese player told me that he was fat because he just didn't like any of the foods that were healthy for him. "Is that really true?" I asked. "You don't like any of them?" I then showed him a list of 50 brain healthy foods, and in fact, he liked about 60 percent of them. The All-or-Nothing ANTs were controlling his food choices and making him fat.

While the country was in lockdown during the pandemic, I heard so many All-or-Nothing ANTs from my patients as well as from people on social media.

Here are 15 examples of All-or-Nothing ANTs, including some of the more common pandemic-induced ANTs I heard:

1. *All of my freedom is being taken away from me during quarantine.*

2. *We're all going to get COVID-19.*

3. *I am not a good father.*

4. *No one cares about me.*

5. *Nothing ever works out for me.*

6. *I am an abject failure.*

7. *I am not a good Christian.*

8. *My boss is taking advantage of me.*

9. *My husband is the devil incarnate.*

10. *We had an argument. I think our relationship is over.*

11. *I couldn't run a mile. I'll never be an athlete and should just quit working out.*

12. *I don't want to talk to anyone anymore.*

13. *My wife never listens to me.*

14. *I thought I did a good report, but my boss asked me to make a few changes. I can't do anything right.*

15. *I'm so bored; there's nothing to do.*

Send the All-or-Nothing ANTs packing.

# LESS-THAN ANTS *(fuel Abandoned, Invisible, Insignificant, Inferior, and Flawed Dragons)*

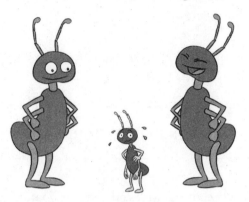

Less-Than ANTs are some of the most toxic ANTs to your self-esteem. Whenever you compare yourself to others in a negative way, these ANTs harass and attack you. They are involved in the epidemic rise of teenage depression and suicide, all exacerbated by social media. Many teens spend hours a day comparing their lives and the way they look to a false sense of others'. Parents can also put unrealistic expectations and pressure on their children to live up to those on the internet. These ANTs come from your Invisible, Insignificant, Inferior, or Flawed Dragons.

Less-Than ANTs usually start with the words "I am not . . ."

1. *I am not good enough.*

2. *I am not a good enough mother/father.*

3. *I am not a good enough daughter/son.*

4. *I am not a good enough wife/husband.*

5. *I am not a good enough boss/employee.*

6. *I am not a good enough Christian.*

7. *I am not a good enough investor.*

8. *I am not smart enough.*

9. *I am not rich enough.*

10. *I am not tall enough.*

11. *I am not strong enough.*

12. *I am not pretty enough.*

13. *I am not funny enough.*

14. *I am not kind enough.*

15. *I am not good enough to be a professor/doctor/lawyer.*

---

*I keep fighting voices in my mind that say I'm not enough.*

**LAUREN DAIGLE, "YOU SAY"**

---

If you continually compete with and compare yourself to others, you'll have lower self-esteem, and you will be bitter. If you compete to be your best self, you will be better. The problem is often we are comparing our behind-the-scenes self with another person's highlight reel.

When I was a young psychiatrist, just out of my training, I noticed that whenever I felt someone had it all together (a great marriage, perfect children, career success, etc.), within three weeks they would be in my office telling me about their troubles, such as a gambling addiction, extramarital affairs, and children who were stealing. I met parents with a criminal record, a priest who no longer believed in God, and so on. It was such an important lesson. Few people are who they show to the outside world. I have had the honor of treating US Senators, Oscar- and Emmy-winning actors, Hall of Fame athletes, Grammy-winning musicians, business leaders, and megachurch pastors. These wonderful people all had the same issues and insecurities as the rest of us.

When you allow the Less-Than ANTs to steal your happiness, your Invisible, Insignificant, Inferior, or Flawed Dragons get stronger. You stop celebrating your wins if you didn't do better than others. You can come to resent the people you love and feel envious when they succeed. On social media, when we compare ourselves to others, we are jealous of the *perception* of their reality and start hating our *actual* reality. Be careful not to fall for the "InstaSham" version of other people's lives.

# JUST-THE-BAD ANTS *(fuel Wounded, Ancestral, Hopeless, Helpless, and Death Dragons)*

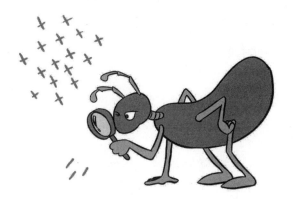

Thousands of years ago, human minds were trained to focus on the negative because it kept people safe. Today, even though lions, tigers, and bears are not likely to eat you, your brain is still primed to pay attention to potential danger before focusing on anything positive.

To take advantage of our negative tendency, internet marketing dragons feed us a nonstop stream of negative news to increase clicks and traffic to their sites. Have you noticed breaking news is pervasive and never good? Our society is infesting us with Just-the-Bad ANTs. These pesky creatures see only the bad in a situation and ignore anything good! Unless you manage your internet usage, you are swamped with distressing news about the coronavirus, terror attacks, nonstop political scandals, fires, floods, hurricanes, global warming, mass shootings, murder-suicides, executions, and more. Negative news sells, and since we are always being sold something for the financial gain of others, we are flooded with toxic thoughts.

Just-the-Bad ANTs also zoom their beady eyes in on your mistakes and problems. They fill your head with failure, frustration, sadness, and fear. So many dragons love to feast on these ANTs. These ANTs can take virtually any positive experience and taint it with negativity. They are the judge, jury, and executioner of any new experiences, new relationships, and new habits. Some examples of Just-the-Bad ANTs include thoughts like these:

1. *Quarantine is the worst.*

2. *The world is more dangerous than ever.*

3. *So many people are dying from COVID-19.*

4. *I went to the gym and did a hard workout, but the guy on the bike next to me was talking the whole time, so I'm never going back there.*

5. *I gave a presentation at work, and even though many people told me they loved it, one person fell asleep during my talk, so it must have really been terrible.*

6. *I only got into the college of my second choice. I failed.*

7. *This pandemic will never end.*

8. *I love people who don't love me back.*

9. *I got together with an old friend, but she showed up ten minutes late for lunch, so I'm not going to call her again.*

10. *I cut back my caffeine intake from ten cups of coffee a day to two, but I wanted to get down to no coffee by now, so I should just quit trying.*

11. *I got into our vacation home an hour late and the lights were out. What a disaster!*

12. *My record debuted at #2 on the* Billboard *charts; I am so disappointed.*

13. *Our city league baseball team finished second; the whole season was a waste of time.*

14. *My son got four As on his report card but also two Bs. I'm so disappointed.*

15. *I've been good with my diet all week, but because I cheated on Friday, it ruined everything.*

I once helped a child who was depressed. In the beginning he could think only about the bad things that had happened to him. He had recently moved nearby and told me he would never have friends (even though he already had several), he would do poorly in his new school (even though he got mostly good grades), and he would never have any fun (even though he lived near the beach and Disneyland). By focusing on the negative, he was making it very hard to adjust to his new home. We worked on noticing what was right more than what was wrong, which helped him feel better.

# GUILT-BEATING ANTS *(fuel Should and Shaming Dragons)*

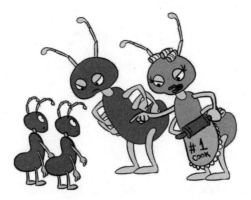

With Guilt-Beating ANTs, motivation comes from moral beatings you received from others, such as parents and authority figures: "You should have done that. You ought to do this. You mustn't think like that ever again." These ANTs have their origin in the Should and Shaming as well as Responsible Dragons from the Past. Whenever you think in words like *should, must, ought,* or *have to,* your brain is beating you up with guilt. Of course, there are things you should and should not do. But trying to motivate behavior with guilt often backfires and can be counterproductive. Here are some examples of Guilt-Beating ANTs:

1. *I'm not a good son because I do not call my dad. I should do better.*

2. *I should Zoom or FaceTime with my parents more often.*

3. *I have to give up sugar.*

4. *I must start counting my calories.*

5. *I ought to exercise more.*

6. *I should be more giving.*

7. *I'm ashamed of the sexual experiences I had as a preteen. I should not have done those things.*

8. *My struggles are my fault. I should be better.* (This is also a Blaming ANT.)

9. *I'm selfish for seeking help. I shouldn't have to do it.* (This is also a Labeling ANT.)

10. *I should quit because all the work problems are my fault.* (This is also a Blaming ANT.)

11. *I feel guilty for taking time for myself.*

12. *I should be able to beat this depression without medicine.*

13. *I should not have made this move to a new job.*

14. *I must do better in school.*

15. *I should be a better wife/husband.*

What happens when you allow these ANTs to circle in your mind? Do they make you more inclined to connect with your parents, cut the sugar, count calories, be physically active, or be more giving? I doubt it. It is human nature to push back when we feel as if we "must" do something, even if it is to our benefit. The key to overcoming Guilt-Beating ANTs and stop feeding the Should and Shaming Dragons is to replace them with phrases such as:

*I want to do this.*

*It fits with my goals to do that.*

*It would be helpful to do this.*

*I want to visit my parents because they are special to me.*

*My goal is to stop eating sugar because it will reduce my cravings; prevent energy crashes, diabetes, and inflammation in my body; and get me off this emotional roller coaster.*

*I want to count my calories because it will help me learn to take control of my eating.*

*It is in my best interest to go to the gym because it will help me feel more energized.*

*I am a giving person, and it is my goal to give more to causes I believe are worthwhile.*

### *Terry: Behavior is more complicated than you think, so don't believe every thought you have*

Terry had a very hard time keeping up in school. His parents and teachers made him believe that he was "lazy, stupid, and irresponsible" (Should and Shaming Dragons). His whole life he felt an incredible amount of shame. He eventually dropped out of school, fell into depression (Hopeless and Helpless Dragons), and lived in isolation. He didn't believe he could ever have a family and worked very hard just to get by. When he was 46, his "mental health" worsened, and he believed there must be something wrong with his brain, but his MRI was normal, which it often is in such cases. MRIs look at the brain's structure, not how the brain functions, which is often the root of the problem.

When he came to our clinic in New York, his SPECT scan showed severe damage to his frontal lobes, which was consistent with a traumatic brain injury he later learned he'd had as a small child. He talked to his mother about the scan, and they cried together for hours. They realized he didn't have a bad attitude; he had a troubled brain.

Terry got serious about rehabilitating his brain using our program, including diet recommendations, supplements, and hyperbaric oxygen therapy. Months later his scans showed dramatic improvement as did his life. His mood, energy, and hope have soared, and he now sees a much brighter future for himself, including the possibility of a family.

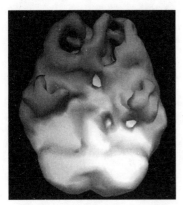
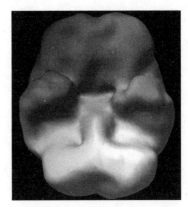

Terry's surface SPECT scan
Before

Terry's surface SPECT scan
After

## LABELING ANTS *(fuel Should, Shaming, and Judgmental Dragons)*

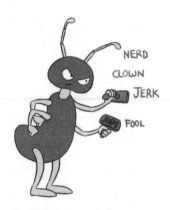

Whenever you label yourself or someone else with a negative term, you inhibit your ability to take an honest look at yourself or someone else. You lump yourself or the other person with everyone else who has that label. Your Should, Shaming, or Judgmental Dragons have taken over.

Labeling ANTs strengthen negative pathways in the brain, making the ruts deeper and their walls thicker. These habitual ruts lead to troubled behaviors. If, for example, you label yourself as "lazy," then why bother trying to do better in school or at work? Labeling ANTs will cause you to give up before you try, and they will keep you stuck in your old ways. Examples of Labeling ANTs include:

1. *I'm a white boy; I don't fit in.* (from someone half Hispanic and half Caucasian)

2. *I'm lazy.*

3. *I'm a loser.*

4. *I'm a lousy businessperson.*

5. *I sound like an idiot.*

6. *I'm fat/short.*

7. *I'm evil because I hurt a cat when I was eight.*

8. *I'm selfish.*

9. *He's a jerk.*

10. *She's weak.*

11. *He sucks.*

12. *You're weird.*

13. *You're too gullible.*

14. *You're a bad son.*

15. *He's a narcissist.*

The problem with Labeling ANTs is that they trick you into thinking that it is impossible to change. You are what you are. But that's not true. You can change your thinking to focus on what's possible:

> *I am capable of so much more than I have given myself credit for. I am going to commit to eating better, exercising more, and spending more time with family and friends.*
>
> *I know I can do better in school if I just apply myself more. I'm going to ask my teacher to help me set up a study plan and show me some time-management skills.*
>
> *I know I can do better at work. I'm going to make a list of my strengths and strategize ways to use them more effectively.*

A word of caution: Even positive labels can be harmful. For example, I tell parents not to praise children for being smart, but rather praise them for working hard. When you tell children they are smart, they become more performance oriented and assume that intelligence cannot be improved. If they start to struggle with a new task, they may feel "not smart" and give up. But if you praise children for working hard, when they come up against a difficult task, they will persist because they "work hard." Special, Spoiled, Entitled, and Responsible Dragons may also feed on Labeling ANTs, filling you with pride so you look down on others. I'm all for affirming yourself and others, but be cautious of going overboard to the detriment of others.

## FORTUNE-TELLING ANTS *(fuel Anxious, Wounded, Hopeless and Helpless Dragons)*

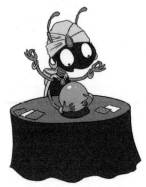

These ANTs predict the worst, and then they make things worse still. Fortune-Telling ANTs are masterful at linking, stacking, and attacking to provide the fuel for anxiety and panic disorders. For instance, look at the progression of ANTs that led Jimmy (from the introduction) to his suicidal thoughts.

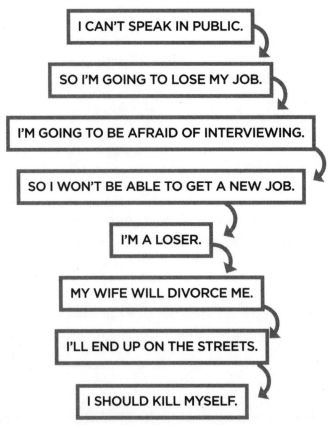

I CAN'T SPEAK IN PUBLIC.

SO I'M GOING TO LOSE MY JOB.

I'M GOING TO BE AFRAID OF INTERVIEWING.

SO I WON'T BE ABLE TO GET A NEW JOB.

I'M A LOSER.

MY WIFE WILL DIVORCE ME.

I'LL END UP ON THE STREETS.

I SHOULD KILL MYSELF.

Don't listen to these lying ANTs! They think they can see what is going to happen in the future, but all they really do is think up bad stuff that makes you upset. They creep into your mind and fill the future with fear. Of course, it is always helpful to prepare for potential problems, but if you spend all your time focused on a fearful future, you will be filled with anxiety. Examples of this deceiver include:

1. *Nothing will ever be "normal" again after the pandemic. Everything will be worse.*

2. *I'm doomed to be unemployed for years.*

3. *Our economy will never recover from the shutdown.*

4. *I'm going to get sick and be on a ventilator.*

5. *I'll become homeless.*

6. *My children will also have a mental illness.*

7. *I'll die without him.*

8. *If I give that presentation, I'll have a panic attack.*

9. *None of my investments will pay off.*

10. *I'll look stupid when I talk.*

11. *I won't be able to buy a house.*

12. *I'll never exercise again.*

13. *I'll never sign up for Toastmasters.*

14. *My friend killed himself; I am doomed.*

15. *My kids will get a better dad if I die.*

Predicting the worst in a situation causes an immediate rise in heart and breathing rates and can make you feel anxious. It can trigger cravings for sugar or refined carbs and make you feel as if you need to eat to calm your anxiety. What makes Fortune-Telling ANTs even worse is that your mind is so powerful it can make what you imagine happen. When you think you will sprain your ankle, for example, that thought may deactivate the cerebellum, making you more clumsy and likely to get hurt. Similarly, if you are convinced you won't get a good night's sleep or find a new relationship, you will be less likely to engage in the behaviors that might make it so. The key to eliminating these ANTs is to talk back to them:

> *If I strengthen my immune system with brain-healthy habits and supplements, it will reduce my chances of getting COVID-19.*
>
> *As long as I stretch and remain focused when I run, I will be fine.*
>
> *I am going to ace that presentation.*
>
> *I am going to make sound, informed financial investments. That way, even if some of them don't work out, I'll still land on my feet.*
>
> *If I can't fall asleep right away, I'll just read a good book until I get tired.*

## MIND-READING ANTS *(fuel Abandoned, Invisible, Insignificant, Inferior, Flawed, and Anxious Dragons)*

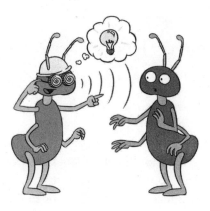

These ANTs are convinced they can see inside someone else's mind and know how others think and feel without even being told. It leads us to tell ourselves things like *Everyone thinks I'm stupid* or *They're laughing at me.* When you're sure you know what others are thinking, even though they have not told you and you have not asked them, Mind-Reading ANTs are infesting your brain.

I have 25 years of education, and I can't tell what anyone else is thinking unless they tell me. A glance in your direction doesn't mean somebody is talking about you or mad at you. I tell people that a negative look from someone else may mean nothing more than that he or she is constipated! You just don't know. Other Mind-Reading ANTs include thoughts like:

1. *My dad thinks I'm weak.*

2. *My boss doesn't like me.*

3. *People think I'm fearful for wearing a mask in public.*

4. *My friends think I won't be able to keep up with them on our hike.*

5. *My father thinks I'll never amount to much.*

6. *People think I'm dumb.*

7. *People think I'm being treated for depression to get attention.*

8. *People at work don't care about me.*

9. *I can die, and people won't care.*

10. *Everyone is disappointed in me.*

11. *My mom doesn't think I measure up compared to my siblings.*

12. *I frustrate all the people who know me.*

13. *My wife would rather be with someone else.*

14. *My pastor doesn't care about me.*

15. *He thinks everyone else is an idiot.*

Remember the 18-40-60 Rule (see page 24)? The vast majority of people spend their days worrying and thinking about themselves, not about you, so stop trying to read their minds. Don't let these ANTs erase your good feelings. When you don't understand something or someone, ask for clarification. Mind-Reading ANTs are infectious and pit your dragons against other people's dragons.

# IF-ONLY AND I'LL-BE-HAPPY-WHEN ANTS
*(fuel Inferior, Flawed, Anxious, Wounded, Should, Shaming, Judgmental, Grief, and Loss Dragons)*

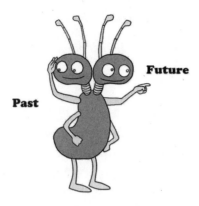

I once heard Byron Katie tell an audience, "Whenever you argue with reality, welcome to hell." I have shared that line many times with my patients. Spending time in regret for things in the past you cannot change leads only to pain and ongoing frustration. Regret manifests itself in "If only . . ." thinking patterns for what occurred and "I'll be happier when . . ." for regrets in the present you hope will change in the future. Each of these phrases ensures self-defeating thoughts because they take you out of the present moment. The other side of regret is unhappiness with the present, hoping for a different future. Here are examples:

1. *If only I had sold my stocks before the coronavirus hit.*

2. *If only my parents had been rich.*

3. *If only I were taller/skinnier/prettier.*

4. *If only I had stayed in school.*

5. *If only I hadn't made that mistake.*

6. *If only I had stopped drinking earlier.*

7. *If only child protective services hadn't taken my kids away from me.*

8. *I'll be happier when I retire.*

9. *I'll be happier when he/she agrees to marry me.*

10. *I'll be happier when our divorce is finalized.*

11. *I'll be happier when I have children.*

12. *I'll be happier when the children are grown and out of my hair.*

13. *I'll be happier when I graduate from college.*

14. *I'll be happier when I land that promotion.*

15. *I'll be happier when I lose 10 pounds.*

These ANTs only waste your time and your gifts. Practice gratitude for what you do have and where you are today because that's all you have. Ask yourself, *Do I have everything I need right now?* This can help ground you in the present and keep you from focusing on regrets about the past or unrealistic expectations of the future.

## BLAMING ANTS *(fuel Special, Spoiled, Entitled, Judgmental, and Ancestral Dragons)*

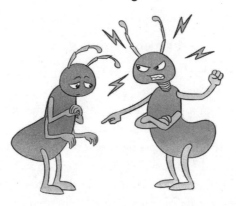

The first and most devastating hallmark of self-sabotage is the tendency to blame others when things go wrong in life. These ANTs often originate with Special, Spoiled, Entitled, or Judgmental Dragons. And Ancestral Dragons come to feed on them. When something goes wrong at work or in their relationships, they often find someone to blame. They rarely recognize their own problems.

The bottom-line statement goes something like this: "If only you had done something differently, I wouldn't be in the predicament I'm in. It's your fault, and I'm not responsible." Blame starts a dangerous downhill slide that goes something like this:

> **BLAMES OTHERS**
> **"IT'S YOUR FAULT."**

> **SEES LIFE AS BEYOND PERSONAL CONTROL**
> **"MY LIFE WOULD BE BETTER IF IT WEREN'T FOR . . ."**

> **FEELS LIKE A VICTIM OF CIRCUMSTANCES**
> **"IF ONLY THAT HADN'T HAPPENED, THEN . . ."**

> **GIVES UP TRYING**
> **"NOTHING WILL EVER GO RIGHT FOR ME. WHY TRY?"**

*Permitting your life to be taken over by another person is like letting the waiter eat your dinner.*

**VERNON HOWARD**

Blaming others temporarily rids yourself of feelings of guilt or responsibility. However, it also reinforces the idea that life is out of your control, that others can determine how life goes for you. This causes much inner turmoil, leading to Anxious and Helpless Dragons.

Psychiatrists have known for some time that the patients who do the worst in psychotherapy are the ones who take no personal responsibility for getting better. In fact, as early as Freud (1927), a major goal of psychotherapy has been increasing patients' sense of personal responsibility. Dr. Carl Rogers went so far as to develop a "personal responsibility" scale to predict those who would get better with treatment and those who would not.

Of all the ANTs, Blaming ANTs are the most toxic. I call them red ANTs because they not only steal your happiness, but they also drain your personal power. When you blame something or someone else for your problems, you become a victim of circumstances who can't do anything to change the situation. Be honest and ask yourself if you have a tendency to say things like:

1. *It's their fault that the coronavirus is still spreading.*

2. *It's your fault I failed because you didn't do enough to help me.*

3. *It's not my fault I eat too much; my mom taught me to clean my plate.*

4. *I'm having trouble meeting this deadline because the client keeps changing his mind. I'm miserable, and it's all his fault!*

5. *My boyfriend didn't call on time, and now it's too late to go to that movie I wanted to see. He's ruined my night!*

6. *My husband did not protect me from the bad decision I made at work.*

7. *It's my boss's fault I did not get promoted.*

8. *It's my child's fault.*

9. *It's the teacher's fault my child is failing.*

10. *It wasn't my fault that I wasn't prepared for the meeting. They never give enough notice.*

11. *That wouldn't have happened if you had been better to me.*

12. *How was I supposed to know the boss wanted the reports in two days? He should have told me.*

13. *It's your fault that you got pregnant; you should have protected yourself.*

14. *If it was so important, why didn't you remind me?*

15. *That's not my job.*

Beginning a sentence with "It is *your* fault that I . . ." can ruin your life. In order to break free from the Blaming ANTs, you have to make it your responsibility to change. It is your life, not anyone else's.

At the same time, self-blame is equally toxic. Self-blame can result from Should, Shaming, or Responsible Dragons. If you are constantly taking the blame whenever someone else gets upset, feels anxious, or is at odds with you, step back to assess what's your responsibility and what isn't. Don't let your dragons or others' dragons put all your focus on self-blame. Always strive to be a good coach to yourself rather than someone who is toxic or abusive.

## HOW CHALLENGING 100 OF YOUR WORST THOUGHTS CAN CHANGE YOUR LIFE

One of the first exercises I give patients is to have them write down 100 of their worst ANTs. Then we subject each of them to the elimination process. If you do this with diligence and thoughtfulness, I promise you will stop feeding your dragons, end self-defeating thoughts, and be more in control of your happiness and destiny. The brain learns by repetition.

Undisciplined or negative thinking is like a bad habit. The more you engage in it, the more easily the ANTs will attack and take over your mind. These bad thinking habits form through a process called long-term potentiation. When neurons fire together, they wire together, and the negative thoughts become an ingrained part of your life. That is why you need to do this exercise 100 times to teach your brain a new, more rational way of thinking.

You do not have to believe every thought you have. If you want emotional freedom, it is critical to develop the skill of guiding and directing your thoughts. This is the first step in developing strong mental discipline. Whenever you feel sad, mad, nervous, or out of control, write down your ANTs, identify which type they are (there may be more than one type), and then ask yourself the simple questions I learned from Byron Katie.[4] They are life-changing. There are no right or wrong answers; they are just questions to open your mind to alternative possibilities. Meditate on each answer to see how it makes you feel. Ask if your stressful thoughts make your life better or worse.

ANT:

ANT Type(s):

**Five Questions**

1. **Is it true?** Sometimes this first question will stop the ANT because you already know it's not true. Sometimes your answer will be "I don't know." If you don't know, then do not act like the negative thought is true. Sometimes you may think or feel that the negative thought is true, but that is why the second question is so important.

2. **Is it absolutely true with 100 percent certainty?**

3. **How do I feel when I believe this thought?**

4. **How would I feel if I couldn't have this thought?**

5. **Turn the thought around to its exact opposite, and then ask if the opposite of the thought is true or even truer than the original thought. Then use this turnaround as a meditation.**

During the pandemic, one of my patients called in a panic because she lost her job, and she told me, "I'll never be able to work again." I guided her through the five questions to work on that thought:

ANT: *I'll never be able to work again.*

ANT Type(s): Fortune-Telling

1. **Is it true?** Yes

2. **Is it absolutely true with 100 percent certainty?** No, I already have part-time work lined up.

3. **How do I feel when I believe this thought?** Trapped, victimized, helpless

4. **How would I feel if I couldn't have this thought?** Massively relieved, happy, joyful, free, like my usual self

5. **Turn the thought around to its exact opposite:** I can get work again. **Any evidence that that's true?** I have valuable skills that will help me get a job.

   **Thought to meditate on:** *I have valuable skills that will help me get a job.*

If you do this exercise with your most toxic thoughts, it will change your life because your brain will begin to stop listening to the negativity running through your head and start listening to the truth. Remember, this is not about positive thinking. It is about accurate thinking. To make this technique clear, here are several more examples:

## FROM A MAN SUFFERING WITH SEVERE DEPRESSION. ONE OF HIS MOST TOXIC ANTs WAS, *I'M GOING TO END UP LIKE MY FATHER WHO ABANDONED US.*

**ANT:** *I'm going to end up like my father who abandoned us.*

**ANT Type(s):** Fortune-Telling

1. **Is it true?** No

2. **Is it absolutely true with 100 percent certainty?** No, I will always be here for my children and wife.

3. **How do I feel when I believe this thought?** Like I lost at life; I feel like a failure, scum, sad, anxious, angry

4. **How would I feel if I couldn't have this thought?** Relieved, free, safe

5. **Turn the thought around to its exact opposite:** I am not going to end up like my father. **Any evidence that that's true?** Yes, I am with my family, employed, and not addicted to drugs.

    **Thought to meditate on:** *I am not going to end up like my father.*

## FROM A WOMAN WHO HAD TO TESTIFY AGAINST A MAN WHO MURDERED HER SON IN A BAR FIGHT

**ANT:** *I'm evil because I want him to suffer.*

**ANT Type(s):** Labeling

1. **Is it true?** No

2. **Is it absolutely true with 100 percent certainty?** No

3. **How do I feel when I believe this thought?** Horrible, like I am a bad person. Who am I to judge others?

4. **How would I feel if I couldn't have this thought?** Still grieving my son but without self-recrimination

5. **Turn the thought around to its exact opposite:** I am not evil; I am loving. I am just going to tell the truth and allow the justice system to work. **Any evidence that that's true?** Yes, I do many helpful and loving things for other people.

    **Thought to meditate on:** *I am loving.*

## FROM A POLICE OFFICER WHO WAS STRESSED AT WORK AND FEELING AS THOUGH HE WAS NOT MAKING A DIFFERENCE

**ANT:** *I'm not making a difference.*

**ANT Type(s):** All-or-Nothing

1. **Is it true?** Yes

2. **Is it absolutely true with 100 percent certainty?** No

3. **How do I feel when I believe this thought?** Useless, weak, withering, sad

4. **How would I feel if I couldn't have this thought?** Optimistic, purposeful, content, motivated, happier

5. **Turn the thought around to its exact opposite:** I am making a difference. **Any evidence that that's true?** Yes, every day I have good interactions that help others.

   **Thought to meditate on:** *I am making a difference.*

## FROM A STATE DEPARTMENT EMPLOYEE WHO WAS STRUGGLING WITH COWORKERS. HE TOLD ME, "THE MORE YOU DO, THE MORE YOU GET SCREWED."

**ANT:** *The more you do, the more you get screwed.*

**ANT Type(s):** Just-the-Bad

1. **Is it true?** Yes

2. **Is it absolutely true with 100 percent certainty?** No

3. **How do I feel when I believe this thought?** Angry, useless, unmotivated

4. **How would I feel if I couldn't have this thought?** Purposeful, happy, more present and in the moment

5. **Turn the thought around to its exact opposite:** The more I do, the less I get screwed. **Any evidence that that's true?** Yes, the more I do, the more I help and live my purpose.

   **Thought to meditate on:** *The more I do, the more I help and live my purpose.*

**FROM A WIDOWED MOTHER OF FOUR CHILDREN WHO WAS CHRONICALLY STRESSED AND UNHAPPY BUT NOT ASKING FOR HELP FROM HER FAMILY. SHE TOLD ME, "I SHOULD BE THE STRONG ONE."**

ANT: *I should be the strong one.*

ANT Type(s): Guilt-Beating

1. Is it true? Yes

2. Is it absolutely true with 100 percent certainty? No. At this pace, I am unable to do it all myself.

3. How do I feel when I believe this thought? Defeated, depressed, overwhelmed, like running away

4. How would I feel if I couldn't have this thought? Like a good mother because I would ask for help and have it when I needed it.

5. Turn the thought around to its exact opposite: I don't have to be the only strong one. I can ask for help. **Any evidence that that's true?** Yes, my family has offered, and I can accept their help with gratitude.

   **Thought to meditate on:** *I can ask for help.*

**TEN EXAMPLES FROM JIMMY, WHO DID THIS EXERCISE SHORTLY AFTER WE MET.**

ANT #1: *I can't speak in public.*

ANT Type(s): Fortune-Telling

1. Is it true? Yes

2. Is it absolutely true with 100 percent certainty? No

3. How do I feel when I believe this thought? Petrified, panicked, ashamed

4. How would I feel if I couldn't have this thought? Confident

5. **Turn the thought around to its exact opposite:** I can speak in public and have done so many times.

   **Thought to meditate on:** *I can speak in public.*

**ANT #2:** *I'd be better off dead.*

**ANT Type(s):** All-or-Nothing, Just-the-Bad

1. **Is it true?** No

2. **Is it absolutely true with 100 percent certainty?** No

3. **How do I feel when I believe this thought?** Suicidal, sad, worthless, hopeless

4. **How would I feel if I couldn't have this thought?** Happier and wanting to be alive

5. **Turn the thought around to its exact opposite:** I'd be better off alive for many reasons, most important of which is to care for my wife and children.

   **Thought to meditate on:** *I am better off alive.*

**ANT #3:** *I will sound like an idiot.*

**ANT Type(s):** Fortune-Telling, Labeling, Less-Than

1. **Is it true?** No

2. **Is it absolutely true with 100 percent certainty?** No

3. **How do I feel when I believe this thought?** Stupid

4. **How would I feel if I couldn't have this thought?** Relaxed, smart

5. **Turn the thought around to its exact opposite:** I will not sound like an idiot, which is why I have been promoted at work and my wife married me.

   **Thought to meditate on:** *I will sound smart.*

**ANT #4:** *I am not as smart as everyone in the room.*

**ANT Type(s):** Less-Than, All-or-Nothing

1. **Is it true?** No

2. **Is it absolutely true with 100 percent certainty?** No

3. **How do I feel when I believe this thought?** Incapable

4. **How would I feel if I couldn't have this thought?** Capable

5. **Turn the thought around to its exact opposite:** I am as smart as everyone in the room. I graduated from college and have a wonderful job.

   **Thought to meditate on:** *I am as smart as everyone in the room.*

**ANT #5:** *I am not a good father because I discipline my children.*

**ANT Type(s):** Less-Than, All-or-Nothing, Guilt-Beating

1. **Is it true?** No

2. **Is it absolutely true with 100 percent certainty?** No

3. **How do I feel when I believe this thought?** Like a bad parent, not as good as others

4. **How would I feel if I couldn't have this thought?** Strong, like a good father

5. **Turn the thought around to its exact opposite:** I am a good father because I discipline my children with love. If I never disciplined my children, they would grow up entitled, which would be bad for them. I strive to be thoughtful when I discipline.

   **Thought to meditate on:** *I am a good father because I discipline my children with love.*

**ANT #6:** *I am weak.*

**ANT Type(s):** Labeling, All-or-Nothing, Just-the-Bad

1. **Is it true?** No

2. **Is it absolutely true with 100 percent certainty?** No

3. **How do I feel when I believe this thought?** Inadequate

4. **How would I feel if I couldn't have this thought?** Confident

5. **Turn the thought around to its exact opposite:** I am not weak. I am a survivor and have grown through intense trauma.

   **Thought to meditate on:** *I am strong.*

**ANT #7:** *I have a mental illness.*

**ANT Type(s):** Labeling

1. **Is it true?** Yes

2. **Is it absolutely true with 100 percent certainty?** No. I have brain health issues that I am working on.

3. **How do I feel when I believe this thought?** Different

4. **How would I feel if I couldn't have this thought?** Normal

5. **Turn the thought around to its exact opposite:** I do not have a mental illness but rather brain-health issues that were never properly treated.

   **Thought to meditate on:** *I have brain-health issues, but who wouldn't with my past? I am working on them every day.*

**ANT #8:** *I am not good enough.*

**ANT Type(s):** Less-Than, All-or-Nothing, Just-the-Bad

1. **Is it true?** No

2. **Is it absolutely true with 100 percent certainty?** No

3. **How do I feel when I believe this thought?** Weak, inferior

4. **How would I feel if I couldn't have this thought?** Free, happy, enough

5. **Turn the thought around to its exact opposite:** I am good enough.

   **Thought to meditate on:** *I am good enough.*

**ANT #9:** *I was given away because I was the worst kid of all.*

**ANT Type(s):** All-or-Nothing, Mind-Reading, Labeling

1. **Is it true?** No

2. **Is it absolutely true with 100 percent certainty?** No

3. **How do I feel when I believe this thought?** Bad

4. **How would I feel if I couldn't have this thought?** Loved

5. **Turn the thought around to its exact opposite:** I was given away because my mother was anxious and overwhelmed, and she thought my grandfather would provide a better life for me since he was a successful businessman.

   **Thought to meditate on:** *My mother was anxious and overwhelmed, and I forgive her for sending me away.*

**ANT #10:** *I'm a "white boy." I don't fit in.*

**ANT Type(s):** Labeling

1. **Is it true?** No

2. **Is it absolutely true with 100 percent certainty?** No

3. **How do I feel when I believe this thought?** Rejected

4. **How would I feel if I couldn't have this thought?** Accepted

5. **Turn the thought around to its exact opposite:** I am not a "white boy." Being half Caucasian and half Hispanic was confusing, but I can relate to both cultures.

   **Thought to meditate on:** *I am unique and can relate to both of my cultures.*

# ELIMINATE BAD HABIT DRAGONS

## IDENTIFY THE AUTOMATIC BEHAVIORS THAT RUIN YOUR LIFE

*Until you make the unconscious conscious, it will direct your life and you will call it fate.*

CARL JUNG

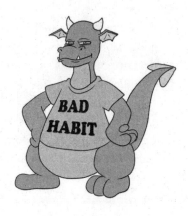

Although your brain is always listening to dragons, habits pretty much run your life. Virtually everything you do is based on a series of habits you've developed over your lifetime. Our daily habits include hundreds of routines, such as saying no to bread; telling your spouse you love her at the end of phone calls; making your spouse an unsweetened, almond milk decaf cappuccino in the morning (I do this for my wife every morning to show her I love her); brushing your teeth; flossing; shaving; blow-drying your hair (not mine); showering; feeding pets; putting away the dishes; closing cabinet doors; taking out the trash; doing the laundry a certain way. Habits are behaviors that have been automated, so we barely need to think about them.

There is a constant dance between your Dragon Tamer (PFC), your amygdala (the part of your emotional brain that responds to threats), and your basal ganglia (where habits are shaped and stored). When the PFC (see section 7 for more on the Dragon Tamer) is healthy and strong, it can help direct and supervise the addition of healthy habits. When it is weak, you are more easily influenced by untamed dragons, and your impulses can take over, causing many bad habits to form. Once formed, good or bad habits take the same amount of energy.

For many people, as the shelter-at-home orders dragged on due to the coronavirus, long-time good habits gave way to bad ones. People who hadn't indulged in bread, cookies, or muffins for years were suddenly baking up a storm. Others who had strong work habits at the office found themselves being distracted, inattentive, and unproductive while trying to work from home. Still others who exercised on a regular basis could no longer motivate themselves to get moving and became couch potatoes. The rampant stress and anxiety of the pandemic weakened Dragon Tamers everywhere and let the Bad Habit Dragons take control.

*When your Dragon Tamer is weak, you are much more likely to be visited by Bad Habit Dragons.*

Some of your habits move your life forward in ways that make you proud, while other habits become dragons that lead to trouble in relationships, work, and finances. Wasting time, allowing distractions, interrupting, arguing, and being disorganized or oblivious are habits that hurt you. Taking your words and actions off autopilot and using your PFC to direct them in a purposeful way will boost your happiness, improve your relationships, and increase your overall success. For example, whenever I go to a restaurant and the waiter asks if I want an alcoholic drink and leaves bread on the table, I am not oblivious to how my response will impact my health. I say no to the alcohol and ask him to take away the bread. My automatic responses are habits; they are stored in a part of the brain called the basal ganglia. Habits are processes that developed over time to either get and stay healthy or get and stay sick.

Telling the waiter no is a "cornerstone habit" that sets up the rest of the meal. Do you know why waiters start with alcohol and bring free bread to the table? Both lower blood flow to the prefrontal cortex (PFC) and weaken the Dragon Tamer. Alcohol directly drops function of the PFC, which is why your decision quality suffers the more you drink. Bread quickly turns to sugar in your stomach, causing an immediate spike in blood sugar and the hormone insulin, which drives tryptophan into the brain. Tryptophan is the precursor to the "don't worry; be happy" neurotransmitter, serotonin, which, like alcohol, lowers blood flow to the PFC, making you more likely to order additional food, including dessert, even when you'd told yourself before the meal that you'd be sensible. I often say to my patients and myself, "Make one decision, not 30." If I make the one decision not to keep the bread on the table, I will not glance at it 30 times and have to make 30 decisions not to eat it.

Most people think of habits as a single task, but they are generally made up of many smaller behaviors (habit stacking), such as saying no to the bread:

Waiter automatically brings bread to the table.

I say, "No, thank you, please take it away."

Waiter often looks surprised and says, "Are you sure? It's really good."

I say, "As sure as I can be."

Two minutes later, the busboy, seeing there is no bread, brings it again.

I say, "Please take it away."

Habits form through a process called long-term potentiation. When neurons fire together, they wire together, and habits and responses become an ingrained part of your life. Long-term potentiation occurs when the brain learns something new, whether it's good or bad for you, and causes networks of brain cells to make new connections. Early in the learning process, the connections are weak (I had to really think about saying no to the bread), but over time, as you repeat behaviors, the networks become stronger, making the behaviors more likely to become automatic, reflexive, or habitual.

---

*Once formed, good habits take the same
amount of energy as bad habits.*

---

What makes something a bad habit? It has a negative impact on your health, relationships, or finances; others find it annoying; and it becomes a dragon that influences your brain. Bad habits can be stopped with training. There are thousands of bad habits. For illustration, we will explore 10 common Bad Habit Dragons that steal your happiness, health, and relationships.

## 10 BAD HABIT DRAGONS (BHD)

1. Saying Yes, When You Should Say No BHD
2. Automatic No or Arguing BHD
3. Interrupting, No-Filter BHD
4. Trouble with the Truth BHD
5. Distracted, Obsessive, Multitasking BHD
6. Procrastinating (I'll Do It Tomorrow) BHD
7. Disorganized BHD
8. Let's Have a Problem BHD
9. Overeating BHD
10. Oblivious BHD

*Convert Bad Habit Dragons into good ones*

You can retrain or convert Bad Habit Dragons into good ones using five simple steps.

1. **Identify the Bad Habit Dragon and start tracking it.** Establish a baseline of the unwanted habit and how often it occurs. This will help you track your progress. Only work on retraining one Bad Habit Dragon at a time for about 30 days. In 10 months, you'll be able to tackle all 10 of these if needed.

2. **Identify the cues or triggers for the habit.** When you notice an urge to do something (e.g., at a restaurant for dinner), ask yourself questions such as:

   • What is the time of day? *Time:* evening
   • Where are you? *Location:* restaurant

- Who are you with? *People:* with my wife or friends
- How are you feeling? *Mood:* generally happy
- What is happening? *Action:* waiter asks about alcohol, leaves bread on table

Answering these five questions will help you know the cues or triggers to the behavior.

3. **What are the rewards or benefits of the behavior?** Know what you are seeking. Is it pleasure, energy, excitement, happiness, relief, relaxation, acceptance, love, or something else?

4. **What are other ways to get the same or better benefits?** How else could you get what you are looking for? Experiment with different options. Whenever you experience a bad habit trigger, substitute something else to see if you can get the same benefit but in a way that will serve your health and happiness rather than hurt it. Only love behaviors that love you back. For example, when you catch yourself wanting to nibble on something at a restaurant, ask for some carrots, cucumber, or celery sticks. You'll get a satisfying crunch.

   Before I got serious about being healthy, I gave in to my urge for bread, especially freshly made bread dripping in butter. Yet when I fell in love with my brain, I realized I love being healthy, having energy and cognitive clarity, and being able to get into the same size jeans I wore in high school much more than the momentary pleasure of unhealthy food. The new benefits were so much better than the old ones. I now see free bread as a "weapon of mass destruction," and I feel badly when I give in to a behavior that does not serve my health.

5. **Build a new routine.** Now that you know the cues and rewards, build a new routine(s) to get what you want (in section 7, you'll create a One Page Miracle to outline your goals). Focus on the rewards you will get without that bad habit. For any habit you want to break, keep it simple. For example:

   1. What is the habit you want to change? Stop nighttime eating

   2. What are the cues to the habit? Evening, after dinner, alone or with friends

3. What rewards are you seeking? *Initial:* Relief from craving and habitual eating patterns (brain craves sameness, whether it is good or bad) *Rewards without this behavior:* Long-term relief from cravings and better control over eating habits

4. What new routine(s) can you build? *After dinner, I will not eat again until midmorning the next day. When cravings surface, I'll drink a glass of water or take a short walk.*

In James Clear's book *Atomic Habits*, he says that to create a new habit, make it obvious, know the cues; make the new habit attractive, give rewards; make it easy, get into a new routine, the simpler the better; and make it satisfying.[1]

## SAYING YES, WHEN YOU SHOULD SAY NO BAD HABIT DRAGONS

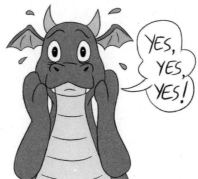

This people-pleasing Bad Habit Dragon overwhelms people and can make them bitter and chronically stressed. Like many bad habits, it is associated with low PFC activity, which limits forethought. When someone asks you to do something, you reflexively say yes without thinking through all the consequences and end up so busy you don't have time for family and other priorities. The Saying Yes, When You Should Say No Bad Habit Dragon has its origins in the Abandoned, Invisible, Insignificant, Anxious, or Should and Shaming Dragons that erroneously believe if you do more for others, they will approve of and like you more.

I once treated Carter, an attorney who told me he didn't have time to work out or eat healthy because he was so busy. When we went through his week, it was clear he had committed himself to many activities that served other people's needs but few of his own. I taught him the magic phrase "I have to think about it." I had him practice saying it over and over in front of the mirror. Then he was to filter every request through this question: *Does this fit the goals I have for my life?* Does it fit his relational goals, work goals, financial goals, or goals for his physical, emotional, or spiritual health? If it didn't, he would politely decline. Over three months, this simple exercise changed his life. He had more time for his wife, children, sleep, and even *pro bono* work, which was one of his goals.

### *Control the Saying Yes, When You Should Say No Bad Habit Dragons*

1. **Do you have this habit?** If you often feel overwhelmed, tired, or have no time for yourself, this dragon is likely biting you. Track it.

2. **What are the cues or triggers?** Trying to please people, impulsively responding, avoiding feelings of guilt.

3. **What are the rewards you get?** *Initial:* Significance, being the good guy or gal, points in heaven. *Rewards without this behavior:* Time for things that matter more.

4. **Build a new routine.** Whenever someone asks you to do something, start by saying, "I have to think about it." Then filter your response through the goals you have. If it doesn't fit, politely decline, but be firm by saying something like "I'm not going to be able to fit that into my schedule." Post "I have to think about it" in at least three places you see daily.

---

*New Routine: "I have to think about it."*
*Ask yourself,* **Does it fit my goals?**

---

# AUTOMATIC NO OR ARGUING BAD HABIT DRAGONS

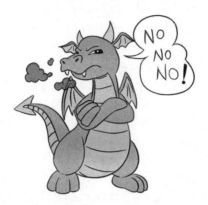

The opposite of the last Bad Habit Dragon, this dragon is stuck in the terrible twos. It is normal for two-year-old children to assert their independence and automatically say no. If I wanted a kiss from one of my kids when they were two, I'd often use reverse psychology and say I didn't want a kiss, which generally worked (don't judge me for being manipulative). Children usually outgrow the automatic no between the ages of three to four. It's cute when they're two, but it's really irritating when they're six, 16, 46, or 86.

Many years ago, I noticed that people who tended to be argumentative or oppositional (automatically say no) had increased activity in the anterior cingulate gyrus (ACG) in the frontal lobes. Think of the ACG as the brain's gear shifter. It is involved with cognitive flexibility, as well as shifting attention, seeing options, and detecting errors. When it works too hard, people tend to listen only to dragons and ANTs. They can worry (fixated on certain thoughts), be rigid or inflexible, hold grudges, see too many errors in themselves and others, and often get stuck on the words *no, no way, never, you can't make me do it.*

My dad had this Bad Habit Dragon and excessive activity in his ACG. Whenever I'd ask him for something, such as permission to borrow the car, the answer was automatically no. My siblings and I knew if we wanted something from Dad, he would first say no, then a week or two later he would think about the request and sometimes change his mind. *No* was his first response.

In 1972, when I turned 18, I had to sign up for the draft because the US was still at war in Vietnam. When I showed interest in joining the Army to become a veterinarian's assistant (I had wanted to become a veterinarian since I was young), my father told me I couldn't do it (his automatic response) because there was a *war* going on. So what did I do? Joined the Army! Three weeks later, I was in basic training at Ford Ord, outside Monterey, California, with my head shaved and people screaming at me, calling me a maggot. Because my dad said I couldn't do it, I had to do it (a normal adolescent process called individuation). If he had said, "That's an interesting idea; let's talk about it," it's likely I would have never been called a maggot.

The Automatic No or Arguing Bad Habit Dragons cause stress to relationships. One man told me that whenever he wanted to make love with his wife, he had to act as if he really didn't want to make love. He said, "If I would ask her directly, she would say no 99 times out of 100. If I would lock our bedroom door at night (a sign that he wanted to be intimate with her), she would become tense and say she wasn't interested. If I acted uninterested, just rubbed her back for a long time, then maybe I would have a chance. The amount of work and planning it took to make it happen often wasn't worth the effort." The automatic no puts a great strain on many relationships.

### Control the Automatic No or Arguing Bad Habit Dragons

1. **Do you have this habit?** If your first response is no, or you start formulating an argument in your head before people have finished their thoughts, you likely have this dragon. Don't automatically say you don't have it—a natural tendency of this dragon. Track it.

2. **What are the cues or triggers?** Whenever someone asks you for something or to do something, or when you are in an emotional conversation.

3. **What are the rewards you get?** *Initial:* Being right, staying in control, having sovereignty over your time and decisions. *Rewards without this behavior:* Improved cooperation and relationships.

4. **Build a new routine.** Before answering questions or responding to requests in a negative way, catch yourself, take a breath, and think first if it's best to say no. Often it's helpful to take a deep breath, just to get extra time before responding. For example, if your spouse asks you to do something, before you say no, take a deep breath and ask yourself if saying no is really in everyone's best interest, if it fits the goals you have for the relationship. In fact, you can use the same

line that I gave for the last dragon: "I have to think about it." The automatic no has ruined many relationships. Take enough time to ask yourself if "no" is really what you want to say.

---

*New Routine: Recognize the automatic tendency to argue or say no, take a deep breath, and ask yourself what response is really in the best interest of the situation and relationship.*

---

## INTERRUPTING, NO-FILTER BAD HABIT DRAGONS

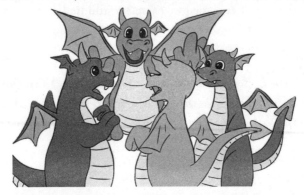

Watch any political talk show, and you'll see and hear these Bad Habit Dragons screaming and talking over each other. They don't really listen; they say the first thing that comes to mind. As soon as someone else says something, the other person is formulating a response without really knowing what the other person is saying. Political pundits do this. Supervisors do this. Many parents do this—and it shuts down communication.

Over the years, many patients have told me that they are brutally honest. I think to myself, *That's usually not helpful.* People with the Interrupting, No-Filter Bad Habit Dragon usually have low activity in their PFC, so they don't filter what they're going to say before they say it. Thinking about the impact your words will have on others before you say them is critical to healthy relationships.

In lectures I often ask audiences, "How many of you are married?" Half the audience will raise their hands. Then I ask, "Is it helpful for you to say everything you think in your marriage?" The audience laughs and collectively says, "No!"

This dragon can be rude, justify its behavior by saying he has to speak up or he'll forget what he was going to say, and tends to dominate conversations. In addition, people with this dragon have trouble waiting in lines. Children and employees often clam up when a parent or supervisor suffers from this Bad Habit Dragon.

Over the years, I've seen many teenagers who were shut down because their parents talked over them, didn't listen, and were constantly telling the teens how to think. That's what happened to Brandon. At 15, he became depressed and rebelled. As soon as he got home from school, he would shut himself in his room and come out only to grab some food. If his parents tried to coax him out of his room, he would lash out, telling them to leave him alone. His parents thought Brandon was the problem and brought him to see me. They told me he was uncommunicative and guaranteed that he wouldn't talk to me. I told the parents to leave Brandon with me.

When it was just the two of us, I let him know that I was there to listen to him, and I gave him the space he needed to express himself. Over time, he opened up and told me that his parents never allowed him to finish a sentence or to share his opinions, so he just gave up trying. That's when I invited his parents to become a part of Brandon's therapy and helped them understand that they were part of the problem and could be part of the solution.

### Control the Interrupting, No-Filter Bad Habit Dragons

1. **Do you have this habit?** Has anyone told you that you interrupt or jump into conversations too quickly? Do people tend to shut down around you? Do you tend to say the first thing that comes to mind without considering the impact your words have on others before you say them, or do you tend to act without thinking?

2. **What are the cues or triggers?** Conversations with people close to you, such as coworkers and friends; when you are intoxicated (stop drinking), hungry, tired, angry, in an argument, or overwhelmed by your partner's words.

3. **What are the rewards you get?** *Initial:* Venting or blowing off steam, relieving stress, getting your point across, feeling the need to be right. *Rewards without this behavior:* More connection, more input, better relationships.

4. **Build a new routine.** There are two antidotes to the Interrupting, No-Filter Bad Habit Dragons that improve communication and overall relationship health: learning to ask, "Then what?" and active listening.

   Before you say something, filter it through the impact it may have on others. I often teach my patients to ask themselves, *If I say this, or if I do this, then what are the consequences? Will it bring me closer to my spouse, improve my relationship with my boss, help my children develop in a responsible way, improve my own health?* The more you filter your words and deeds through what you really want, the less "brutally honest" you will be.

---

*New Routine: Think,* **Then what?** *before you say anything.*

---

Active listening dramatically improves communication; most psychotherapists teach this skill. It shuts down the voice of any dragon. It is simple and goes like this:

Step 1: Listen and do not interrupt, no matter how much you get the urge.

Step 2. Repeat back what you hear: "I hear you saying . . ."

Step 3: Listen for the feelings behind what you're hearing: "Sounds like you are feeling frustrated."

Step 4: Listen to the person's response carefully and reflect it back again.

Active listening forces you to pay attention and stops you from thinking about what you're going to say next so you can hear the other person. The rewards are that it increases communication, immediately clears up misunderstandings, and cools down conflicts. When people feel heard, they can often talk through and solve their own problems. When people don't feel heard, or when someone talks over them, it can trigger Abandoned, Invisible, or Insignificant Dragons, as well as Angry Dragons. Active listening can miraculously change relationships in a short period of time.

---

*New routine: Active listening—"I hear you saying . . ."*

---

# TROUBLE WITH THE TRUTH BAD HABIT DRAGONS

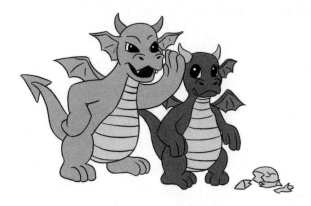

This is a sneaky Bad Habit Dragon. Lying leads to mistrust in your relationships, and if you can lie to others, you also lie to yourself. Of course, you do not need to be brutally honest. I often tell my patients there are ways to say things and there are more tactful ways to say things. Lying is a common bad habit. In fact, according to one study, most people lie once or twice a day.[2] People lie for many different reasons, including:

- To avoid being punished (Anxious Dragons)
- To protect oneself (Wounded Dragons)
- To avoid disappointing others (Anxious Dragons)
- To avoid embarrassment (Should and Shaming Dragons)
- To obtain a reward they did not earn (Spoiled Dragons)
- To promote oneself (Insignificant Dragons)
- To protect another person from being punished (Responsible Dragons)
- To get out of an uncomfortable social situation (Anxious Dragons)
- To exercise power over others (Angry Dragons)

Lying can even ruin your health. One study found that 81 percent of patients lie to their doctors in at least one of seven scenarios: not adhering to prescription medication as instructed, not exercising regularly or at all, not understanding a doctor's instructions, disagreeing with a doctor's recommendations, maintaining an unhealthy diet, taking a specific medication, and taking someone else's medication.[3] It's nearly impossible for you to get the help you need if you're not honest with your caregivers.

There is a difference between "normal" liars—those of us who tell harmless little white lies—and pathological liars.

**Normal liars:**

Give compliments that are not 100 percent genuine

Tell people they're doing well, when they really aren't

Say they are busy to avoid others

**Pathological liars:**

Lie habitually, even when there is no clear benefit

Lie to make themselves look like the hero or victim, and the stories they tell are dramatic, complicated, and detailed

Get a thrill from getting away with it

Tell more lies per day than a normal liar tells

Tend to be younger, male, and have higher occupational status—bad news for hedge fund managers, attorneys, and doctors

Lie the most to their partners and children

Believe lying is acceptable; aren't deterred by guilt or risk of exposure

More likely to lie for their own self-interest, such as to protect a secret

---

# When Children Lie

As a child psychiatrist, I've been teaching parent training for many years. One of the first steps in the program is to have parents post a few rules at home to guide and direct behavior. Rule number one is "Tell the Truth." One of the best gifts you can give children is to teach them to be honest, which builds trust in relationships. Plus, if they can be honest with others, they are more likely to be honest with themselves. So when they tell a lie to get out of trouble, they get a consequence for the wrong act and another one for lying. The rule is very clear: Tell the truth! This includes little lies and big ones. I've found that when you allow a child to get away with the little lies, the bigger ones are easier to tell. Of course, this means if you want children to follow this rule, you cannot tell lies. Children do what you do, not what you tell them to do. When someone calls when you do not want to talk, do not tell your child to lie for you and say you aren't home. That teaches kids that lying is okay.

When lying is a problem, I teach parents an exercise called Truth Training, which begins by identifying lying as a problem to be solved, rather than an indictment on the child's character.

Remember when I told my mother a lie at age six, she cried and told me she never thought she would have a child who would go to hell. Don't do that. Tell the child why lying is a problem—people will not trust them—and tell them you are going to ask them questions you already know the answer to. If they answer honestly, you will be very happy and give them a small reward, such as extra time together, and if they lie, there will be a consequence, such as extra chores. Do it in a matter-of-fact way, without emotion, and always root for them to tell the truth.

---

I'd be lying if I said lying is an easy habit to break.

### Control the Trouble with the Truth Bad Habit Dragons

1. **Do you have this habit?** Track how many times you lie today and in a typical week.

2. **What are the cues or triggers?** When you feel trapped, when you don't want to hurt someone's feelings, or when you hate the truth.

3. **What are the rewards you get?** *Initial:* Which of the reasons people lie (see previous page) apply to you? *Rewards without this behavior:* Feel better about yourself, remember facts more clearly, less stress.

4. **Build a new routine.** See lying as a problem, not an indictment of your character. First, immediately stop lying to your health-care professionals. I often tell my patients their number-one job in healing is to tell me the truth; otherwise, we are wasting everyone's time and their money. When you catch yourself starting to lie, take a breath, pause, and say, "I meant . . ." followed by the truth.

   Journal your lies to stay aware of them. Your self-esteem will go up when your lies go down.

   If you cannot stop, get professional help. You may have ADHD or something brain-related clouding your judgment.

---

*New Routine: When you catch yourself starting to lie, take a breath and say, "I meant . . ." followed by the truth.*

---

# DISTRACTED, OBSESSIVE, MULTITASKING BAD HABIT DRAGONS

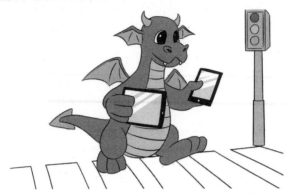

Smartphones, laptops, tablets, email, text messages, the internet, and streaming services are stealing our time and attention often because of the Scheming Dragons on these platforms (see section 5). Many people are not only watching TV, but they are also on other devices at the same time. Technology companies are constantly creating addictive gadgets that hook our attention and distract us from meaningful relationships. Many people are on their phones at mealtimes rather than interacting with family members. A 2015 study found that teens actually spend more time on entertainment media (average nine hours) than they do asleep; tweens are online six hours a day.[4]

Technology has hijacked developing brains with potentially serious consequences for many. As video-game and technology usage go up, so do obesity and depression.[5] Ian Bogost, famed video-game designer (*Cow Clicker* and *Cruel 2 B Kind*) and chair of media studies and professor of interactive computing at Georgia Institute of Technology, calls the wave of new habit-forming technologies "the cigarette of this century" and warns of their equally addictive and potentially destructive side effects.[6]

As part of the gadget revolution, disturbing research from Microsoft reported that humans lose concentration after about eight seconds, while the lowly goldfish loses its focus after about nine seconds.[7] It seems like evolution may be going in the wrong direction. In 2000, the human attention span average was estimated at 12 seconds, which is not great; but losing a third of our attention span in 15 years is alarming![8]

According to an article in the *Harvard Business Review*, "Beware the Busy Manager,"[9] our unhealthy lifestyles are diminishing our capacity at work. Only 10 percent of managers are high in both focus and energy, two of the main ingredients for success. The authors found that 20 percent were disengaged, 30 percent were high in procrastination, and 40 percent were easily distracted. This means that 90 percent of managers, and likely the rest of us, lack focus and/or energy.

### *Beware the Busy Manager*

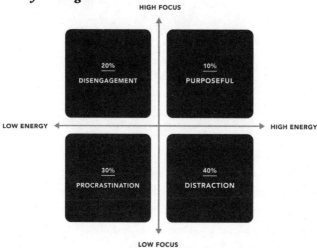

### *Control the Distracted, Obsessive, Multitasking Bad Habit Dragons*

1. **Do you have this habit?** Track how many times an hour you are distracted.

2. **What are the cues or triggers?** Being bombarded by phone calls, emails, texts, etc.

3. **What are the rewards you get?** *Initial:* Satisfy your addiction of having to know what's next or having to distract yourself with entertainment so you don't have to face problems. *Rewards without this behavior:* More time, less stress, better focus.

4. **Build a new routine.** When you need to get things done, shut down your email and put your phone on airplane mode. Your productivity will go way up. Try AppDetox to help stop your phone from distracting you.

---

*New Routine: When you need to get things done, shut down your email and put your phone on airplane mode.*

---

# PROCRASTINATING (I'LL DO IT TOMORROW) BAD HABIT DRAGONS

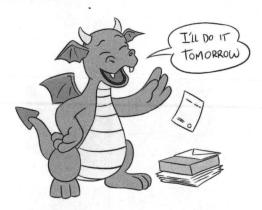

Procrastination is the act of unnecessarily postponing decisions or actions. When you wait until the very last minute to get things done (completing schoolwork, paperwork, or chores; paying bills; buying birthday, anniversary, or Christmas gifts, etc.), it increases stress and often irritates those around you who feel the need to pick up the loose pieces.

If it isn't the last minute, this dragon cannot kick its brain into gear to get its work done. Many parents have told me about the constant fights they have with their children or teens about starting projects early and working on them over time, rather than the night before. Many adults have told me they never did term papers in school or they used amphetamines the night before a due date. Procrastination leads to poorly done, incomplete, or unfinished work.

Procrastination is a hallmark of the ADHD Dragon where your Dragon Tamer (PFC) is not as strong as it could be. Procrastination is also associated with abstract goals, depression, perfectionism, never feeling as though you can get something just right, fear of failure, and low energy.

### *Control the Procrastinating (I'll Do It Tomorrow) Bad Habit Dragons*

1. **Do you have this habit?** Track how many times today you procrastinated or said or thought, "I'll do it tomorrow."

2. **What are the cues or triggers?** You are faced with a task or a decision, but you would rather do something else.

3. **What are the rewards you get?** *Initial:* Don't have to expend energy and effort; can stay in the present moment; receive immediate

gratification rather than future rewards. *Rewards without this behavior:* Get more done with less stress and do a better job.

4. **Build a new routine.** As with lying, don't see procrastination as a character problem but rather as a problem to solve. The secret to stop procrastinating is to have a method to get things done. I use one that is just a few simple steps:

**Know what you want:** Most things in my life start with that question. What are your goals? Write them down and look at them every day. Make sure you create the One Page Miracle on pages 258-259. The first things I look at each day are my One Page Miracle and my to-do and stop-doing lists. Don't try to do too many things at once or little will get done, which is why I also have a stop-doing list. Tim Cook, CEO of Apple, says, "We say no to good ideas every day. We do this to make great ideas happen."[10]

**Have a one- to three-minute huddle with yourself** at the beginning of every day. At Amen Clinics, one of our habits is a daily huddle, where the teams meet for a few minutes each morning to review what happened the day before and what our goals are for the day, all in the context of our overall goals. The huddles keep us in a rhythm of getting things done. Having a brief huddle with yourself will significantly increase your productivity. Decide what you want to accomplish that day in the overall context of your life. Write down three things you want to accomplish that day, and start with the most important one.

**Do the most important things first.** There's a reason dessert is at the end of the meal. If you eat it first, you won't get the nutrition you need. Stop eating dessert first with your time—get the most important tasks of the day done when your energy is highest.

**Do the fewest activities to reach your goal.** Achieving your goals is like trying to move a giant rock. It's not a question of effort but of having the right tools and plan. What tools do you need to get the task done? The right food, exercise clothes, financial tracking tools? Make sure you have those before you expend effort. For example, I schedule exercise rather than leave it up to "when I have time." If I schedule it, no one can take it from me. I also put my walking clothes out the night before so they are ready to go in the morning, and I wear a Fitbit to make sure I am constantly reminded to get enough exercise. Just putting on my watch nudges me to exercise.

**Bundle things you love to do with things you tend to procrastinate about.** For example, listen to podcasts or audiobooks while exercising, or watch your favorite television show while doing household chores. Most mornings, as I am walking, I'm also on a conference call with two of my work teams.

**Give yourself a reward.** Tell yourself that after you finish a difficult task, you'll reward yourself with something special, such as a new book, a warm bath, or a cup of hot tea.

If you find you cannot stop procrastinating using these simple steps, make sure you do not have ADHD interfering with your life. See page 256.

---

*New Routine: The secret to stop procrastinating is to have a method to get things done.*

---

# DISORGANIZED BAD HABIT DRAGONS

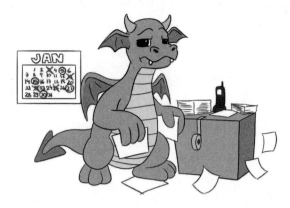

Through a series of Bad Habit Dragons (Saying Yes, When You Should Say No; Distracted, Obsessive, Multitasking; Procrastinating [I'll Do It Tomorrow]) or being overloaded, many people struggle with organization, both for time and their space. They tend to be late, finish tasks at the last moment, or have trouble completing tasks on time. They also tend to struggle keeping their spaces tidy, especially their rooms, book bags, filing cabinets, drawers, closets, and paperwork.

Nothing is more frustrating to a boss, coworker, family member—anyone—than to be waiting on someone who is poorly organized, unprepared for their daily tasks, or late. You've probably felt the irritation of waiting for someone to finish a task later than planned or changing plans because of somebody's poor organization. It can linger for some time, as it did for Billie's boss.

Billie was a bright, articulate, and energetic administrative assistant. She rose quickly in a small computer company because of her verbal skills. Yet her disorganization became a glaring problem when her boss promoted her to office manager. The smooth-running operation began to sputter as she ignored many of the small details. At first Billie's boss was going to fire her for her deficiencies. After he talked to a consultant, however, he realized that he had promoted Billie because of the abilities she showed in the previous position but that they had little to do with what he expected from her in her current one. Instead of firing her, he sent her to several "organizational" workshops, and she dramatically improved.

Psychiatrists say that people who are chronically unprepared for tasks or always late to appointments are manifesting underlying hostility. They get their anger out in passive-aggressive ways; instead of telling someone they're mad, they act it out by being late or sabotaging their tasks. Being disorganized and chronically late is also a hallmark sign of ADHD. When there is low activity in the PFC, it is harder to be organized and on time.

---

*Organizing is what you do before you do something, so that when you do it, it's not all mixed up.*

**CHRISTOPHER ROBIN, A. A. MILNE'S *WINNIE THE POOH***

---

### Control the Disorganized Bad Habit Dragons

1. **Do you have this habit?** How are your room, desk, purse, closets, drawers? How is your timeliness? What would your partner or parents say about your organization?

2. **What are the cues or triggers?** Being in a hurry; not devoting time to organize your day, tasks, or space; overloaded schedule; high stress; too many distractions.

3. **What are the rewards you get?** *Initial:* You believe it saves you time. *Rewards without this behavior:* You will save much more time in the long run by being more efficient.

4. **Build a new routine.** Ask for help from a friend or family member who is organized. Or hire a professional organizer to come to your home or work to teach you systems and to organize your spaces. Then make sure he or she comes back monthly to help you build the new habits. Here are a few more organizational tips:

**Schedule similar tasks together,** such as errands, appointments, maintenance, or phone calls.

**Spend your time doing things that are consistent with your goals.** Keep a to-do list of the important tasks you need to get done today, this week, and in the near future. Update this list as necessary. Relying on this list is more accurate than relying on your memory. If possible, schedule your most important activities for the hours when you are at your peak. Learn to say no. Make a list of what not to spend your time doing and keep it in front of you as a handy reminder. Cut unwanted calls short. Unsolicited calls waste a lot of time. I often start conversations by saying something like "I only have a minute . . ." End calls that are taking too much time with something like "I need to pick up this other call" or "I have an appointment" (even if the appointment is only with yourself).

**Watch out for the great time thieves:** These include procrastination, indecisiveness, regrets, fear of failure, worry, and distraction. Don't get distracted by low-value activities, such as social media, binge-watching series on Netflix, or playing video games.

**Be prepared for gifts of time.** Always carry some work or relaxing things to do with you for times when you may have to wait, such as before doctors' appointments, in traffic jams, on an airplane, or on a commuter train. Use the time to your advantage by listening to podcasts or audiobooks, writing notes or letters, creating a menu or grocery list, or tackling any other small task that's already on your to-do list. Change your perception of these moments from dead or wasted time to productive time for you.

---

*New Routine: Ask for help from a friend, family member, or professional to teach you systems and to organize your spaces.*

---

## LET'S HAVE A PROBLEM BAD HABIT DRAGONS

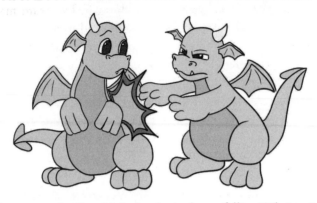

Do you know people who think the sky is always falling? Their minds habitually go to the worst possible outcome, and they express it to others. They frequently say negative things, or they constantly stir up trouble. I call this automatic tendency the Let's Have a Problem Bad Habit Dragon. I first noticed it in one of my ADHD patients. She started every psychotherapy session by talking about how she was going to kill herself. She noticed this made me anxious and seemed to enjoy telling me the gruesome details of her plan. After about a year of listening to her, I finally realized she wasn't really going to kill herself. She was using my reaction as a source of stimulation. After getting to know her very well, I told her, "I don't think you want to kill yourself. You love your four children, and I can't believe you would ever abandon them or model suicide as a way for adults to handle problems. I think you use these stories as a way to stimulate your brain. Without knowing it, your ADHD causes you to play the game of 'Let's have a problem.' This ruins any joy you could have in your life." (Don't try this at home.) Initially, she was very upset with me (another source of conflict, I told her), but she trusted me enough to at least look at the behavior. Decreasing this Bad Habit Dragon and the need for turmoil became one of our goals together and helped her over time.

I've noticed this Bad Habit Dragon in many other ADHD patients but also in those who have had concussions (injuring the PFC), in people who didn't get much sleep (causing low blood flow to the PFC), and in those who had undisciplined minds. Without enough stimulation to the PFC, the brain looks for ways to increase its own activity. Being upset, angry, or negative acts as a stimulant that increases the fight-or-flight neurotransmitter adrenaline, which increases your heart rate, blood pressure, and muscle tension, just as a cup of coffee or a bit of cocaine does.

People with the Let's Have a Problem Bad Habit Dragon often pick on others to get a rise out of them or make them upset. It is unconscious behavior, and they are often not aware they are doing it. I've heard many times from parents of ADHD children, "If we have a bad morning at home, our child has a good day at school" (the yelling and fighting stimulated them), or "If we have a good morning at home, he had a bad day at school" (there was no stimulation, so the child picked on other kids or the teacher). So often, family members of my patients with this dragon say, "I'm so tired of fighting with my brother [sister, mother, father, son, daughter, etc.]. Why does there have to be this turmoil? It seems as if they cannot be happy with peaceful coexistence. They have to fight."

Rosemary and Chrissy, mother and 16-year-old daughter, constantly fought. It didn't seem to matter whether it was about anything specific. It could be curfew, clothes, music, tone of voice, whatever. Chrissy was struggling in school, and her parents brought her to our clinic for evaluation. During the initial interview with Chrissy and her mother and father, I watched the two females go after each other. The tone between them was contentious, mutually irritating, and on edge. The father told me to watch their interactions. He said, "This is how they live at home. Everything is an issue. Everything is a problem. They both hold on to their own positions and cannot let go. It's as if they have to irritate each other. I often don't want to come home because I know I'll have to listen to their battles." Both Chrissy and Rosemary were diagnosed with ADHD. After I balanced their brains, the tension diminished dramatically as did the father's stress level.[11]

### Control the Let's Have a Problem Bad Habit Dragons

1. **Do you have this habit?** Do you tend to find the negative wherever you look or stir up trouble for no particular reason? One morning, after I made breakfast for my wife and nieces, I asked how they liked it. Tana said it was good. "Only good?" I asked. My Let's Have a Problem Dragon was lashing out. When people give you a compliment, do you find a way to diminish it? Some examples:

   "You look pretty today."
   "Didn't I look pretty yesterday?"

   "We did great in business this month."
   "What happened last month?"

   "I got all As and one B."
   "What's with the B?"

"My book was a *New York Times* bestseller for three weeks."

"Well, it's not close to those that were on the bestseller list for three years."

2. **What are the cues or triggers?** Waking up; being around others; feeling bored.

3. **What are the rewards you get?** *Initial:* Express your unhappiness to get it out of your head. *Rewards without this behavior:* Less stress, better relationships.

4. **Build a new routine.** Before you say anything negative, ask yourself if the negativity serves your relationships or your own mental health. *Does it fit the goals I have for my life or this relationship? Does it fit?* are three powerful words to help break the pattern of negativity or conflict-seeking behavior.

---

*New Routine: Ask yourself,* **Does the negativity fit the goals I have for my life or this relationship? Does it fit?**

---

## OVEREATING BAD HABIT DRAGONS

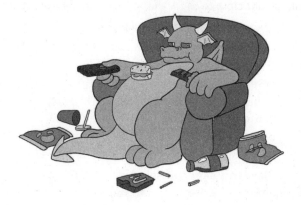

Nearly everywhere you go (schools, work, shopping malls, movie theaters, airports, ballparks, etc.), someone is trying to sell you food that will kill you early and that feeds the Overeating Bad Habit Dragon. The Standard American Diet (SAD) is filled with pro-inflammatory foods that increase your risk for diabetes, hypertension, heart disease, cancer, ADHD, depression, dementia, and obesity, which is now a serious national crisis with 72 percent of Americans overweight and 40 percent obese.[12] I've been writing and teaching about this for decades now. Many published studies, including two of my own, report that as your weight goes up, the size and function of your brain go down.

Karissa wanted to lose weight, but her brain was constantly listening to temptations and giving in. On her way to work, she couldn't pass the Krispy Kreme shop without stopping to pick up a couple of Glazed Lemon Filled doughnuts. When she went to the movies with her boyfriend, the aroma of buttered popcorn was so intoxicating that she had to get a large tub. And whenever she went to visit her mom who lived in a nursing home, she couldn't resist stopping at the See's Candies shop next door. Karissa had an Overeating Bad Habit Dragon that was driving her behavior and hurting her brain.

The excessive fat on your body is not innocuous. It disrupts your hormones, stores toxins, and produces chemicals that increase inflammation. This is the biggest brain drain in US history and is now a national security crisis as up to 71 percent of young applicants for the military are rejected because they are unfit for duty.[13] When obesity is combined with diabetes, which I call "diabesity," the risk is worse. High blood sugar levels damage your blood vessels.

Our weight problem is not just an adult issue. In children ages 2 to 19, obesity has increased from 13.9 percent in 1999–2000 to 18.5 percent in

2015–2016.[14] Food scientists and fast food companies are targeting your kids with weapons of mass destruction, which I define as foods that are highly processed, pesticide sprayed, artificially colored and sweetened, high in sugars, low in fiber, food-like but not real, laden with hormones, and tainted with antibiotics.

Don't let this dragon hijack your brain and your relationships. It'll ruin your health and invite a host of other dragons to the party.

### Control the Overeating Bad Habit Dragons

1. **Do you have this habit?** If you are overweight, obese, or have little control over your eating behavior, you live with this dragon.

2. **What are the cues or triggers?** Notice what is happening around you—for some strange reason, whenever I pass a Jack-in-the-Box, my brain wants an iced tea and a chicken fajita sandwich, which is not the worst thing in the world, but it's certainly not the best.

   Time of day—know your vulnerable times. Morning, lunch, midafternoon, dinnertime, late night? Many people who overeat at night are not hungry in the morning. Location also matters. Whenever I go to a movie theatre and smell the pro-inflammatory popcorn raised with pesticides and cooked in unhealthy oils, the smell triggers the desire for it, even though I know better.

   Being with specific people or at specific places can trigger cravings if you tend to eat certain foods or get drinks with them. For me, my mom's house was one of them. When I made the decision to get healthy, I would eat something healthy before I went to her home, so my Overeating Bad Habit Dragon was under control.

   Many people use food to change their moods. Carbohydrate-laden foods boost serotonin and help calm the brain's emotional centers, which is why people get addicted to doughnuts, cupcakes, cookies, and bread.

3. **What are the rewards you get?** *Initial:* Satisfy cravings, enjoy the designer foods to get an explosion of flavor. *Rewards without this behavior:* Leaner, smarter, happier, healthier, and longer life.

4. **Build a new routine.** Your brain already has a food routine—is it serving you or hurting you? If it is not serving you, create a new one. Here's mine:

Breakfast: either eggs and organic blueberries or a healthy shake around 10 a.m. (I do 12 to 16 hours of intermittent fasting most days)

Snack: fresh-cut veggies with mashed avocados or an apple and almonds

Lunch: salad with grilled veggies and a protein, such as chicken or lamb

Afternoon snack: nuts and fruit

Dinner: protein and veggies

Dessert: sugar-free dark chocolate or fruit

The trick is to find foods you love that love you back and schedule them into your meals. Make a list of foods you like that fit within the following five simple brain-healthy rules for eating:

- Eat high-quality calories and not too many of them. I think of calories like money. Overspend and your health will become bankrupt.

- Eat clean protein at every meal to balance your blood sugar and decrease cravings.

- Focus your diet on healthy fats from fish, nuts, seeds, and avocados. Fat is essential for brain health.

- When you feel hungry, first drink a glass of water to make sure you were not really thirsty.

- Eat smart carbohydrates that do not raise your blood sugar, such as those found in colorful fruits and vegetables; and limit sugar and carbs that quickly turn to sugar, such as bread, pasta, potatoes, and rice. I call these dumb carbs because they're pro-inflammatory and studies show they can decrease IQ.

- Liberally use brain-healthy spices, especially pepper, cinnamon, nutmeg, garlic, cloves, and turmeric.

To fend off cravings, focus on the biology of decision-making: Know what you want (to be at a healthy weight), keep your blood sugar stable (eat small portions of protein and healthy fat at each meal), make sure to get seven to eight hours of sleep at night, limit alcohol, and limit low-quality foods that quickly turn to sugar, such as bread, pasta, potatoes, rice, and sugar. Planning your food is critical. The payoff is that your Dragon Tamer (PFC) gets stronger and healthier at the same time. Your decision-making improves and you start taking control of your life.

# OBLIVIOUS BAD HABIT DRAGONS

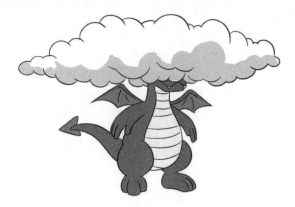

I start many of my lectures with a terrifying video of two women who became trapped on an 80-foot-high railroad bridge with a freight train barreling toward them. Obviously, the train surprised them as they walked along the tracks. Ultimately, the women survived by lying down flat in the middle of the tracks. I show the video because it reminds me of how blind most people are to the health of their brains. If you know brain-health troubles are coming, would you get out of the way? Or would you be like these two women, oblivious to the pitfalls of walking on a railway bridge with no escape?

The Oblivious Bad Habit Dragon (overeating, putting toxic products on your body, never thinking about the health of your brain and body) is likely the worst of all the Bad Habit Dragons. It is where you just don't think about the consequences of your behavior before you engage in it. This is what happens when you let your brain run on autopilot, listening to the loudest dragons, ANTs, and scheming influences (see section 5). In this case, your brain is *not* listening to what it needs to stay healthy. This Bad Habit Dragon is killing us as a society—rates of hypertension, diabesity, depression, and obesity are skyrocketing. Seventy-five percent of health-care dollars in the United States are spent on chronic, preventable illnesses.[16]

### Control the Oblivious Bad Habit Dragons

1. **Do you have this habit?** The dragon is biting you if you do not have a sense of your calorie intake each day; if you do not read food labels; if you do not read personal or cleaning product labels; if you do not know the water quality in your neighborhood.

2. **What are the cues or triggers?** Almost any decision in your day.

3. **What are the rewards you get?** *Initial:* Being oblivious is easy and doesn't require any thinking. *Rewards without this behavior:* Health, energy, longevity.

4. **Build a new routine.** Before you buy anything, do anything, or say anything, ask yourself, *Is this good for my brain or bad for it?* Repeat it over and over until this question becomes a habit itself. Start getting serious about being well and learn what's good for you and your brain. See my book *The End of Mental Illness* for ways to prevent or treat the risk factors that steal your mind and simple strategies to boost overall brain health.

---

*New Routine: Before you buy anything, do anything, or say anything, ask yourself, Is this good for my brain or bad for it?*

---

By now it should be clear that the Oblivious Bad Habit Dragon takes over when the Dragon Tamer is drowsy or asleep. The truth is that all Bad Habit Dragons sneak in while the PFC is off duty or distracted. And then they hurt the capabilities of your Dragon Tamer even more, whispering lies that leave you more vulnerable to the Dragons of the Past and other dragons, not to mention the Scheming Dragons constantly working to profit off you. In our technologically advanced world, we are prey to dragons that generations before us never had to fight off. It's just one more realm where you desperately need a Dragon Tamer that's ready for the battle.

## The Little Lies That Steal Your Health

How you think dramatically affects how you feel and every decision you make. Over the years, I have seen that the "little lies" the Overeating and Oblivious Bad Habit Dragons tell you—and you repeat—are often the gateway thoughts to obesity and illness. Here are some of the common lies I hear in my office:[15]

*Little Lie #1: Everything in moderation.* Just a little can't hurt. I call this one the gateway thought to illness because it is an excuse to avoid making the best decisions for your health.

*Little Lie #2: My memory is no good; that is normal.* Many people start struggling with their memory in their thirties and forties because of poor health habits. It is never normal to have a poor memory; it is a sign your brain needs help.

*Little Lie #3: Getting healthy is too hard.* Being sick is much harder.

*Little Lie #4: I don't want to deprive myself.* Doesn't eating bad food deprive you of your health, your most precious resource? What is worth more? Energy, a trim waistline, health, or the mountain of fries, sodas, cakes, cookies, and the like you have consumed over the last decade?

*Little Lie #5: I can't eat healthy because I travel.* I am always amused by this one because I travel a lot. It just takes a little forethought and planning.

*Little Lie #6: My whole family is overweight [diabetic, addicted, depressed, anxious, etc.]; it is in my genes.* This is one of the biggest little lies. Genes account for only about 20 to 30 percent of your health. Bad decisions drive the vast majority of health problems.

*Little Lie #7: I can't afford to get healthy. Good food is expensive.* Being sick is always more expensive than getting healthy.

*Little Lie #8: I can't find the time to work out.* With a sharper mind, you will actually save time if you work out.

*Little Lie #9: It's Easter, Memorial Day, Fourth of July, Labor Day, Thanksgiving, Christmas, Monday, Tuesday, Wednesday, Thursday, Friday, Saturday, or Sunday.* There is always an excuse to hurt yourself. When you stop believing this little lie, the quality of your decisions and your health will go way up.

*Little Lie #10: I'll start tomorrow!* Unfortunately, tomorrow never comes.

*Little Lie #11: They only serve bad food at work.* Then bring your own food to work. A little planning goes a long way.

*Little Lie #12: I'd rather get Alzheimer's disease, cancer, or diabetes than get rid of sugar.* Unfortunately, this little lie comes from an addiction to sugar and ignorance of the serious consequences of these illnesses.

*Little Lie #13. I'm sad because now that I am getting healthy, I won't do the same things with my kids/grandkids.* Create new activities and a new routine. Instead of baking cookies or holiday pies, make healthy smoothies together or create your own day camp activities.

# OUTFOX THE SCHEMING DRAGONS

## THE IMPACT OF ADVERTISERS, FOOD COMPANIES, GADGETS, NEWS, AND SOCIAL MEDIA

---

*"Deception may give us what we want for the present, but it will always take it away in the end."*

RACHEL HAWTHORNE

---

Even when you identify and tame the Dragons from the Past; the They, Them, and Other Dragons; and the Bad Habit Dragons, the Scheming Dragons will still assault you. We live in a time when Scheming Dragons are on the loose. They are everywhere, deviously sending you messages that feed your dragons and make you fat, depressed, and feebleminded. There are the foot-long hot dogs at the ballpark, the huge meal portions at restaurants, the food pushers who ask us to supersize everything for less money, and the billboards hyping monster foods that will kill you early.

I was once driving north on the 405 freeway in Los Angeles when I saw a billboard for a huge Tower of Torta fast food sandwich from a chain of service stations.

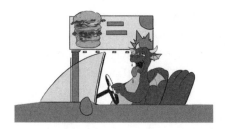

As I turned my head to the other side of the freeway, I saw a billboard with the message "Lose Weight with Lap Band." *Oh great*, I thought, *corporations are encouraging my inner child to make really bad decisions about food for their profit, and as a way to fix the problem, other corporations will offer belly surgery to help me regain control.* The irony seemed pretty crazy.

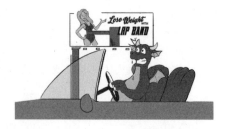

Scheming Dragons are everywhere, trying to make money off your impulses, even if in the near future, it fuels your Anxious, Angry, Inferior, Flawed, or Bad Habit Dragons; makes you depressed or forgetful; and impacts the four circles of your health. And they are using sophisticated neuroscience to get you hooked on whatever they're selling. They capitalize on the latest research on habits and addiction to make your brain crave their products and services and to automate their use, so you don't even think about what you're doing. You mindlessly munch Hot Cheetos until you feel sick and bloated (biological circle), don't notice that you've spent hours going through your social media feed or watching distressing news programs with the latest frightening updates on the pandemic (social circle), and are shocked when you get your credit card statement and see that you've gone way over budget with online purchases you don't even remember making (psychological circle).

In his book *Hooked: How to Build Habit-Forming Products*,[1] author Nir Eyal offers a blueprint of the four-step process the Scheming Dragons use to get you hooked:

- **A trigger starts the process.** An external trigger, such as a pop-up ad, email alert, or TV commercial, pushes you to engage in a behavior. Or an internal trigger, such as boredom or anxiety, prompts you to do something.

- **You take action to get a reward.** You do something because you expect something in return that will make you feel good—a tasty treat, a fun game, or a new outfit.

- **The reward you get isn't always the same.** In the fifties, psychologist and behaviorist B. F. Skinner performed research that found when rewards from an activity are unpredictable, it leads to more compulsive behaviors.[2] More recent neuroscience shows that variable rewards boost the release of the addiction chemical dopamine. Casinos take advantage of this science—think about slot machines, which give variable rewards and are the casino game most often linked to gambling addiction.[3]

- **You engage with the product or service to make it easier to use.** This can be as simple as adding Hot Cheetos to your autoship list, turning on the notifications and alerts for your social-media sites so you won't miss out on anything, or using filters for your sizes or preferences at your favorite shopping sites.

These four steps create a system that makes it easier and easier for you to use the products and services until you're hooked, and it becomes a habit that you don't have to think about.

In this section, we will look at five Scheming Dragons that are on the loose in our society, working to hook you into habits and addictions that will make them rich while doing you harm.

---

*Scheming Dragons hook you into habits and addictions*
*that will make them rich while doing you harm.*

---

## FIVE SCHEMING DRAGONS

1. Food Pusher Dragons
2. Substance and Toxin Pusher Dragons
3. Digital Dragons
4. Contact Sports Dragons
5. Holiday Dragons

### How to outfox the Scheming Dragons

Fight back against the Scheming Dragons with these five simple steps:

1. **Recognize the Scheming Dragons.** Before you mindlessly act on the alerts, texts, emails, ads, package designs, and other triggers that prompt you to take action, stop to ask yourself the following:

   - *Is this more beneficial for me or more beneficial for them?* Scheming Dragons typically entice you to take actions that might help you in the short-term but will benefit them in the long run.
   - *Is this good for my brain or bad for my brain?* Scheming Dragons typically want to rope you into things that are bad for your brain.
   - *Why do I want to take action? Am I really just feeling lonely, bored, or stressed?* If so, look for alternative healthy ways to alleviate those internal triggers.

2. **Look past the messenger.** Scheming Dragons disguise themselves by letting people you trust or admire—celebrities, actors, athletes, social media influencers, news anchors, and attractive models—or creative packaging deliver their messages to you. Always ask who or what is behind the messenger.

3. **Get the whole picture before acting.** Scheming Dragons give you only the tiny bits of information that are most likely to prompt you to buy their product or use their service. They intentionally omit other important facts that might dissuade you from doing so. Make sure to get all the facts first.

4. **Don't make it easier for the Scheming Dragons to hook you.** Don't play into their game by teaming up with them through subscriptions, coupons, games, discounts, and alerts or notifications.

5. **Limit exposure to Scheming Dragons.** Set limits on social media usage and news consumption, avoid places such as fast food joints, and mute ads.

**Examples:**

1. I'm hungry while at the grocery store and see a "health" bar with "all-natural" and "zero carbs" on the label. Sounds good, but I remind myself that many food manufacturers are Scheming Dragons.

2. I look past the messenger and the eye-catching package design and remember there's a corporation behind the product.

3. I read the label to get all the facts. Yikes! It's full of pro-inflammatory oils, artificial sweeteners, and unhealthy chemicals. The "health" bar label should really read "early death," but, of course, that wouldn't boost sales.

4. I don't buy the bar, and I don't sign up to follow them on social media to get three free bars.

5. I vow to *always* read the food labels.

## FOOD PUSHER DRAGONS

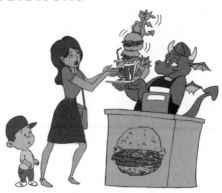

It's nearly impossible to avoid Food Pusher Dragons. They are everywhere trying to entice you to eat food that will steal your focus, make you feel sluggish, put you on a mood roller coaster, and trigger your Bad Habit Dragons. Even at the start of the pandemic, when most of these places were off-limits, the Food Pusher Dragons found new ways to hook you as grocery stores, restaurants, and bakeries promised to deliver the addictive fare you craved. The Standard American Diet (SAD) is filled with foods—or food-like substances—that are largely devoid of nutrients and increase your risk for physical, mental, and cognitive health issues.

Food manufacturing corporations don't try to hide the fact that they purposely make their junk foods addictive. Just think of that Lay's Potato Chips advertising campaign that proudly claimed, "Betcha can't eat just one!" They were right. Junk food giants rely on food scientists to expertly engineer snack items with just the right amounts of unhealthy ingredients to create the perfect combination of flavors and texture to overwhelm the brain to its "bliss point." It's like a hit of cocaine, which activates the brain's reward system and makes you want more, more, more! This is one of the reasons people say they love ice cream, chips, cake, and French fries, and they can't imagine giving them up. They are not eating to live; they are eating to feed their Addicted Dragons that were artificially created for a profit motive.

No food of any kind belongs in the same emotional place in your brain as the love you have for your spouse, children, or grandchildren. Many ancient warriors considered dependence on anything, especially food, a weakness and totally unacceptable. They ate to win; their survival depended on it. I want you to do the same thing if you truly love yourself, your health, your loved ones, and future generations.

Huge corporations are also targeting your children and grandchildren. When a clown or a king with a billion-dollar bankroll can come into your living room and bribe your children with toys to eat low-quality foods that promote illness and early death, it's time to fight back. According to a recent study, the toys fast food companies use to entice children are highly effective weapons in hooking their developing brains to want more of what will hurt their health.[4]

Plus, the companies that produce these unhealthy foods also use adult neuroscience tricks to hijack brains. They purposefully connect gorgeous, scantily clad women to poor-quality food to hook your pleasure centers, somehow making the illogical connection that if you eat those foods, these women will want you or you will look like them. You must know there's no way these beautiful women would look the way they do if their diet regularly consisted of cheeseburgers dripping mayonnaise, mustard, and ketchup down their blouses.

They also use famous actors, singers, and professional athletes to hook you into eating and drinking their health disasters by making you think that their products in some way helped these superstars reach the top of their fields. In commercials, Beyoncé famously sipped Pepsi, Kristen Wiig chomped on a Pizza Hut slice, Peter Dinklage (*Game of Thrones*) and Morgan Freeman rapped about Doritos and Mountain Dew in a 2018 Super Bowl ad, and LeBron James chugs Powerade on the sidelines during basketball games. Do you really think these people hit the big time by consuming sugary sodas, energy drinks, and pizza?[5] Probably not.

Ironically, at the same time many Americans are obsessed with getting healthier. Spending on health and wellness hit a staggering $168 billion in 2017 in the United States,[6] and we've helped the weight-loss industry grow to $72 billion.[7] With all that spending, why are Americans getting fatter and sicker, dying younger, and experiencing more illness than people in other wealthy nations, despite spending nearly twice as much on health care per person?[8] Something's wrong.

In part, it's due to Food Pusher Dragons peddling "health" foods, playing on your desire to get well by offering easy but harmful solutions. They're the ones promising shortcuts—rapid weight loss from fad diets, quick-fix fitness solutions, and "health" foods that that are actually junk food in disguise. For example, certain fad diets might help you lose a few pounds in the short run, but they don't teach you how to eat for long-term brain and body health. Some hard-core fitness trends and gadgets actually put you at increased risk of injury. How is that helping you reach your goals?

Then there are all those so-called health foods. Walk down the aisles of the grocery store, and you'll see products labeled *gluten-free*, *low carb*, *sugar-free*, *vegan*, *all natural*, or some other trendy buzzword. If you're health-conscious, you may be trying to avoid gluten, refined carbs, and added sugars, so these products seem like good choices. But the Food Pusher "Health" Dragons are simply using these catchphrases to grab your attention and prompt you to impulsively put their product in your shopping cart. They're hoping you won't take the time to read the nutrition label and realize that their products are detrimental to your brain and body. Sugar-free? That may be schemer talk for "full of artificial sweeteners." Vegan? That can be the schemer's way of saying, "highly processed, nonfood substance." And gluten-free? That's the schemer's attempt to convince you that cake mix with artificial preservatives, food coloring, and pro-inflammatory ingredients is healthy. It isn't.

I was on vacation a few years ago with my son Antony, and we were shopping together when he put a "healthy" protein bar in our cart. We then looked at the food label, and it had 14 different types of sugar in it, along with artificial dyes and sweeteners!

You also need to watch out for the inadvertent food pushers—the do-gooders who are actually doing the wrong thing by plying you with harmful foods. Think of the receptionist who puts a bowl of candy on her desk at work, the school bake sales, and the doughnuts at church services. (One good thing that may have come out of the coronavirus pandemic is an end—or at least a temporary pause—to these long-standing practices.) Additionally, well-meaning organizations, such as the Girl Scouts, enlist young girls to sell unhealthy cookies as a way to fund their activities. They get you to feel like you're doing something good when you're really just filling your body with sugar, vegetable oil, partially hydrogenated fats, and artificial preservatives that promote disease and mess with your mental wellness.

*Food Pusher Dragon Consequences:* When your brain gives in to the Food Pusher Dragons who are selling food-like substances, it means you're fueling your brain and body with the ingredients that lead to obesity/diabesity (biological circle), as well as Anxious, Hopeless, ADHD, and Overeating Dragons (psychological circle). These food-like substances also shrink your hippocampus (biological circle), one of the major memory structures in the brain, which is associated with an increased risk of dementia.

On the other hand, if your brain is listening to the Food Pusher "Health" Dragons, you may think you're eating a healthy diet when you're actually eating pro-inflammatory foods that will keep weight on and put you at risk for the same problems (biological and psychological circles). When you don't reach your health goals, you're also more likely to feel depressed and trigger the Hopeless and Helpless Dragons (psychological circle). In some cases, these Scheming Dragons convince you to take your health efforts too far. They amp up your Anxious or Inferior Dragons to heighten your worries about eating the wrong thing. This may lead to orthorexia, an excessive obsession with healthy eating that is associated with feelings of anxiety, guilt, and shame.

### How to outfox the Food Pusher Dragons

1. **Recognize the Food Pusher Dragons.** Are they trying to get you to buy their food products? Are they offering a quick fix for a complex problem? Ask yourself if they are good for your brain or bad for it before you buy.

2. **Look past the messenger.** Forget about the gorgeous model, actor, or Girl Scout; think about who is actually selling the food item. Is it someone who is looking out for your health or their bottom line? Don't fall for the idea that someone's product will make you look like the person in the ad.

3. **Get the whole picture before acting.** Read all food labels. Use common sense. A shortcut is not a long-term solution.

4. **Don't make it easier for the Food Pusher Dragons to hook you.** Don't sign up to receive notifications about deals and specials or subscribe to their YouTube channel.

5. **Limit exposure to Food Pusher Dragons.** Avoid the aisles in the middle of the store with the packaged food and stick to the outside. Eat something healthy before you go grocery shopping, so you are not tempted by the impulse buys at the checkout stands or in the "health food" aisles.

## SUBSTANCE AND TOXIN PUSHER DRAGONS

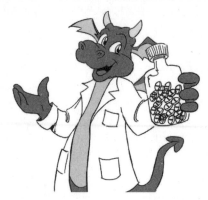

Your brain is the most metabolically active organ in your body. Even though it is only 2 percent of your body's weight, it uses 20 to 30 percent of the calories you consume and 20 percent of the blood flow and oxygen. Exposure to any dangerous substance can damage your brain and your life.

Now, when you think of drug pushers, you probably think of some back-alley dope dealer. But there are many kinds of Substance Pusher Dragons who are selling drugs that can have negative consequences on brain health. Physicians are now prescribing legalized marijuana and CBD (cannabidiol, one of the ingredients of the marijuana and hemp plants) oil to treat symptoms of anxiety, depression, irritability, and aggression even though there's a scarcity of scientific research on it. At the start of the pandemic, when anxiety levels skyrocketed, some states deemed dispensaries "essential businesses," and marijuana sales reportedly increased by 30 percent in Oregon.[9] This could be a case of Substance Pusher Dragons promoting short-term solutions that create long-term problems. Over the last 30 years, I've seen thousands of SPECT scans of patients who were regular marijuana users. In 2016, my colleagues and I published a study on more than 1,000 marijuana users and showed that virtually every area of the brain was lower in blood flow compared to healthy scans, especially in the hippocampus, one of the brain's major memory centers.[10] In 2018, we published the world's largest brain-imaging study on 62,454 SPECT scans to look at how the brain ages. Marijuana was associated with accelerated aging in the brain.[11] So think about your brain health before rushing to your local dispensary.

Substance Pusher Dragons also try to hook you into buying alcohol by spinning science to make it seem like alcohol is a health food. In fact, a 2018 report found that one of the biggest ongoing studies on the effects of moderate drinking as part of a healthy diet was largely funded by—you guessed it—the alcohol industry.[12] Does that sound like good science? For years, even the American Cancer Society seemed to be pushing alcohol with its weak guidelines for cancer prevention: "If you drink alcoholic beverages, limit consumption."[13] This was in spite of the fact that this same organization reports on its website that "Alcohol use is one of the most important preventable risk factors for cancer, along with tobacco use and excess body weight." It wasn't until June 2020 that the ACS finally got more serious and revised its guidelines to say, "It is best not to drink alcohol."[14]

That major news came amidst the pandemic when social isolation had led to feelings of loneliness, stress, depression, and anxiety, prompting a growing number of people who turned to "quarantinis" and Zoom happy hours for a buzz and quick relief from their symptoms. In fact, weekly retail sales of alcoholic beverages soared by 25 to 55 percent during the pandemic.[15] When it comes to the brain, alcohol does not appear to be the health food the alcohol industry would like you to believe. All forms of liquor can impair your cognitive function (biological circle), negatively impact your psychological well-being, and lead to substance abuse (start of social circle problems) in some people.

Some of the slickest Scheming Dragons of all time can be found in the nicotine and tobacco industry. Their advertising messages were so effective that Congress banned airing cigarette ads on TV and radio in 1970. Now, some 50 years later, the Scheming Dragons of the nicotine business are back at it by marketing vaping as a "healthy" alternative to smoking. Juul, the best-known e-cigarette brand, spent $1 million marketing its products on social media and YouTube and had an entire department dedicated to influencer marketing, according to the Truth Initiative.[16] It worked. Vaping is on the rise with twice the number of teens vaping in 2018 compared to 2017.[17] The US Surgeon General has called e-cigarette vaping among youth an epidemic, and as of 2019, over 2,000 cases of serious lung illness along with 39 deaths were due to vaping.[18]

Substance Pusher Dragons also try to hook you on prescription drugs. Think of all those TV commercials you see for medications to treat all sorts of conditions—some you haven't even heard of. The pharmaceutical industry is one of the biggest spenders when it comes to advertising. Their ads play on your emotions by depicting how their little pill can help someone with a debilitating condition quickly transform into a joyful person—walking their dog in nature, dancing with a loved one, or cuddling a grandchild. They make it seem that a pill is all you need to overcome your symptoms. While these heartwarming images continue to roll, you hear a rapid-fire rundown of all the nasty potential side effects—diarrhea, constipation, fatigue, headache, blurry vision, muscle pain, depression, suicidal thoughts. And, oh yeah, death. But these schemers know that 50 percent of the human brain is dedicated to vision, so the images of the happy people stick in our brains, not the list of side effects we hear. As shelter-at-home orders dragged on during the pandemic, new prescriptions for antianxiety and antidepressant medications jumped by 38 percent and 19 percent, respectively.[19] Demand rose so dramatically it actually led to a shortage in the supply of Zoloft and its generic version, sertraline.[20]

Many patients ask for medications by name that they've seen on TV. Take Bridget, for example, who was a sophomore in college when she came to see me. She had been suffering from bipolar disorder for several years and was taking a brand-name prescription she had asked her primary care physician to prescribe. The drug wasn't working for her; she was still suffering from unpleasant symptoms. When we scanned Bridget's brain, it became clear that the root cause of her symptoms was actually an underlying traumatic brain injury. It turned out that she had fallen off a horse when she was 15 years old, and her symptoms had started not long after that. The drug Bridget had been taking wasn't helping her at all and might have been making her symptoms worse. Be careful what you ask for.

Besides drugs, alcohol, and smoking, many other substances are toxic to your brain, such as mold exposure from water damage and heavy metals, including mercury, aluminum, and lead. Did you know when the government took lead out of gasoline, they left it in small airplane fuel? We did a study on 100 pilots and found 70 percent had toxic-looking brains. In a study of 33 well-known brands of lipstick sold in the United States, lead was found in 60 percent of them.[21] Be careful who you kiss, or it could be the kiss of death.

If I handed you a product and told you it could cause fatigue, depression, brain fog, ADHD, memory problems, or psychotic behavior, would you want to use it? Of course not! But Toxin Pusher Dragons are constantly selling products filled with a host of chemicals, pesticides, and fumes that poison the human brain, causing these issues and many more. And tens of millions of Americans are buying them, consuming them, and slathering them on their bodies every day. That's because Toxin Pusher Dragons are exceptionally skilled at making you think you're buying something that is good for you—something that will enhance your health, kill the germs that can cause illness, or make you look younger. And these dragons are everywhere.

## Other Toxins

Carbon monoxide, chemotherapy, and radiation (as they kill cancer cells, they also kill healthy cells) are also toxic to your brain and body. While no schemer is trying to subject you to these substances, exposure to them is just as concerning as having a genetic risk or head trauma. So be even more serious about taking care of your brain.

Toxin Pusher Dragons are in your local grocery store where you least expect them. In the produce section, which is the place where you are supposed to find fresh, nutrient-dense brain-health foods, many toxic bombs are lurking. Mixed in with the good-for-you organic produce are bright shiny apples, plump strawberries, and even dark green kale that have some of the highest pesticide levels. Head over to the fish counter where you think you're making a smart food choice, and you'll find that the schemers are selling fish pumped full of artificial dyes and that have high levels of mercury. Toxin Pusher Dragons also rule the household cleaner aisles. Cleaning agents promise to kill germs, make surfaces sparkle, and do it all with fresh scents. The real story is that regular household cleaners are chock-full of potentially harmful chemicals (including fragrance).

Some of the biggest and baddest Toxin Pusher Dragons are the ones that promise to make you look more attractive and more youthful. The cosmetics, perfume, and toiletries industry spent over $21 billion on advertising in 2020 to entice us to spray, squirt, and smudge more of their products on our faces, hair, and bodies.[22] But the chemicals in many of these products that claim to make us more beautiful can do something very ugly inside our bodies and brains.

*Substance and Toxin Pusher Dragons Consequences:* When your brain is always listening to the Substance and Toxin Pusher Dragons, it can lead to the misguided belief that a substance or pill alone can solve your health issues, clean your house, or make you look and feel better (psychological circle). These substances and products, whether directly damaging or secretly damaging, can give you brain fog, anxiety, depression, and memory loss, and set you up for addiction (psychological circle).

### *How to outfox the Substance and Toxin Pusher Dragons*

1. **Recognize the Substance and Toxin Pusher Dragons.** Are they offering you a substance as an easy solution for your issues? Are they making something seem healthy when you know it probably isn't? To decrease your toxic risk:

   - Limit your exposure whenever you can.
   - Don't opt for short-term solutions (think alcohol and marijuana) that can lead to long-term problems.
   - Buy organic to decrease pesticides and chemical exposures.
   - Read labels! If a product lists ingredients such as phthalates, parabens, or aluminum, don't buy it. What goes on your body, goes in your body and affects your brain.

   Understand that most regular household cleaners and personal care products contain some toxins.

2. **Look past the messenger.** Know who is really behind the information you're getting. Is it the pharmaceutical company or manufacturer?

3. **Get the whole picture before acting.** Do some research. Read the labels. Scan your personal products with the Healthy Living app or visit the Environmental Working Group for healthy cleaning products (ewg.org/guides/cleaners), clean foods (ewg.org/foodscores), the Dirty Dozen list of produce with the highest levels of pesticides (ewg.org/foodnews/dirty-dozen.php), and for safer personal care products (ewg.org/skindeep). Check seafoodwatch.org for safe fish choices.

4. **Don't make it easier for the Substance and Toxin Pusher Dragons to hook you.** Don't start taking or using anything that may be hard to stop. Don't sign up for coupons or free offers for products that contain toxins.

5. **Limit exposure to Substance and Toxin Pusher Dragons.** Say no to alcohol, smoking, and drugs. Stay away from people who are using or offering these substances. Turn off or mute ads.

Stick to safe products. Plus, support the four organs of detoxification: your kidneys, gut, skin, and liver. Boost their ability to clean out your system by drinking plenty of water, eating plenty of fiber, sweating with exercise and saunas (a recent study showed that people who took the most saunas had the lowest risk of memory problems),[23] and eating brassicas, which are detoxifying vegetables, such as broccoli, cauliflower, cabbage, and brussels sprouts.

## DIGITAL DRAGONS

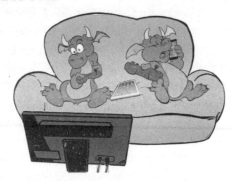

Digital Dragons—technology companies, video-game developers, app creators, news companies, social networks, entertainment providers, and porn sites—have hijacked our brains, stolen our attention, and hooked us on their gadgets, games, and streaming services. Want proof? Just walk into any airport, restaurant, workplace, or school—or your own living room—and see how many people are staring at their smartphones, tablets, or a TV screen. The numbers don't lie. More than 164 million Americans play video games. Netflix jumped to 183 million subscribers worldwide thanks to an additional 16 million who signed up during stay-at-home orders when the pandemic hit,[24] and over 10 million people signed up for the Disney+ streaming service on its first day of operation in 2019.[25]

The Digital Dragons are winning the war for your attention by using a laundry list of proven marketing strategies—scarcity (like Snapchat's disappearing posts), personalization (recommendations tailored to your interests), reciprocity (giving your personal information in order to gain access to their service), and social proof (likes and comments)—to motivate you to become a compulsive user. They also tap into your desire to be part of a group and capitalize on the fear of missing out, or FOMO, the anxiety that comes from the feeling that you've been left out of a fun event or opportunity. What makes the Digital Dragons so frighteningly effective at roping you in is the lightning-fast speed with which they tighten their hold on you.

Do you reach for your phone first thing in the morning to check what awful things have happened in the world overnight? Do you check news websites throughout the day to stay on top of the latest scary developments? News flash: The News Monger Dragons have sucked you into their grasp. News outlets run 24-7 and repeatedly pour toxic thoughts into our brains, making us see impending terror or disaster around every corner to boost their ratings. The constant frightening images activate the brain's fear circuits (amygdala), making us feel chronically anxious and afraid. Information is like crack. Brain-imaging research in a 2019 issue of *Proceedings of the National Academy of Sciences* found that information triggers the dopamine-fueled reward system in the same way as food, money, or even drugs.[26] The authors suggest this neural mechanism explains why we are susceptible to clickbait.

News Monger Dragons tap into the neuroscience that shows the human brain is wired for negativity and pays attention to things that might harm us. That's why they highlight the most sensational crime stories, the latest possible health scares, the juiciest political scandals, and the scariest natural disasters that *might* happen. They say it's to keep you informed and prepared, but it's actually to keep you hooked to their channels or websites.

In 2020, more people than ever fell into this trap as the coronavirus dominated the news. During the pandemic when people were stuck at home, network news viewership skyrocketed, with a 47 percent boost for NBC's *Nightly News*, a 38 percent rise for ABC's *World News Tonight,* and a 31 percent bump for CBS's *Evening News*, according to Nielsen.[27] My anxious patient Brady was glued to the news to hear the latest updates on the virus and signed up for breaking news alerts from several media outlets, so his phone was constantly beeping and feeding him the latest frightening statistics. The onslaught of terrifying news pushed him into a state of panic, which is when he reached out to me. After helping him overcome his panic attack, I explained how to outfox the News Monger Dragons to help prevent future attacks and greatly reduce his anxiety levels.

The schemers in the video gaming industry actually hire neuroscientists to help engineer games that encourage compulsive play. They also use many of the same tactics seen in Las Vegas casinos—variable and intermittent rewards, simplicity, and ease of reentry to the game (think of how easy it is to play a slot machine and to play again if you lose). Others, such as multiplayer games, capitalize on FOMO by allowing others to continue playing when one player logs out. And they entice you to spend real dollars for add-ons and "loot boxes," virtual treasure chests that might contain something useful for the game.

At Amen Clinics, we have treated many teens and adults with video-game addictions, including many who became violent whenever parents put limits on play. We once scanned the brain of a 14-year-old boy who broke the furniture in his room when his parents told him to stop playing. We scanned him after he had stopped playing for a month, and then again while he was playing the game. The scans were so different; it was like we were looking at two different people. The video games caused unhealthy activity in his left temporal lobe, a region of the brain often associated with violence. When he quit playing video games, his brain looked so much better, and he was one of the politest young men I've ever met. What a difference!

The latest newcomers to the Digital Dragon brigade are streaming services that make binge-watching way too easy. Just as one episode of a show is ending, the next one automatically cues up, and before you can decide to turn it off and do something meaningful with your life or go to bed to get the sleep you need, the new episode launches. The next thing you know, it's 2 a.m. and your alarm is set to go off at 6 a.m. These schemers prompt you to tune in with email newsletters and on-screen recommendations based on your viewing habits, and they prey on internal triggers like depression, anxiety, loneliness, and boredom. Streaming services are the ideal way for people to feel like they're escaping Dragons from the Past and other dragons.

Some of the sneakiest Scheming Dragons are the ones behind the social media platforms that steal our time. These days, more than two billion people worldwide use social networks. How do they get you hooked? To keep you scrolling, posting, and commenting, social media outlets have become masterful at using psychological warfare.

These apps are free to join and available at your fingertips. And they have never-ending feeds that refresh constantly, keeping you in a perpetual state of FOMO. They also play a numbers game. As the number of your followers or "likes" goes up, it triggers a release of feel-good dopamine and fires up the reward center in your brain. Research has shown that it's harder for people to resist checking social media than to say no to cigarettes or alcohol.[28]

What's really happening behind the scenes is this: Social Media Dragons need your eyeballs on their advertisers' ads. The more time you spend on your feed, the better for them and the worse for you. Unfortunately, these networks and the social media influencers who have major followings create shame as teenagers and adults endlessly compare themselves to those online who appear to "have it all." Self-esteem takes a serious hit when your life doesn't measure up to all the awesomeness you see online.

Did you know that 12 percent of all websites and 35 percent of all internet downloads are pornographic? Pornography Dragons promise gratification for your most secret sexual desires, and they do it by offering easy accessibility, affordability, and anonymity. The Scheming Dragons of the pornography industry know that men's and women's brains are different when it comes to sexual imagery. They take advantage of brain-imaging research showing that an area of the brain that controls emotions and motivation is much more activated in men than women when viewing sexual material.[29] That's why they tempt men with a never-ending stream of graphic images of nude bodies.

The Pornography Dragons also know that women tend to respond more to emotional intimacy, so they have developed female-friendly erotic material that focuses more on relationships. The number of men and women watching pornography is rising, with a 2014 study reporting that 46 percent of men and 16 percent of women ages 18 to 39 intentionally viewed pornography in a given week.[30]

Pornography Dragons make it so easy to watch pornography because they want people to become compulsive users, spending hours online and losing the ability to control their viewing habits. Research has found that internet pornography addiction shares the same underlying neural mechanisms as substance abuse.[31] Our brain-imaging work on patients who met the criteria for sexual addiction showed that 67 percent had low activity in the PFC (associated with impulse control problems) and 50 percent had too much activity in the anterior cingulate gyrus (associated with a tendency to get stuck on thoughts or behaviors).

*Digital Dragon Consequences:* When your brain is always listening to the distressing News Monger Dragons, it increases anxiety, depression, and stress (psychological circle). In a survey from the American Psychological Association, 56 percent of people said that regularly following the news causes stress.[32] Over time, elevated stress hormones shrink the major memory centers in your brain, increase inflammation, and put excessive fat around your waist (biological circle).

If news isn't what hooks you, but video games and other technology do, as your usage goes up, so does addiction and "gaming disorder" (a condition recognized by the World Health Organization since 2019), anxiety and mood disorders, insomnia, inattention, impulsivity, forgetfulness (all in the psychological circle), and relationship woes (social circle). A 2018 review of brain-imaging studies on gamers found that people with gaming disorder have similar changes to the brain's reward system as those with substance abuse (biological circle).[33] These changes tend to increase impulsivity and impair emotional regulation (biological and psychological circles).

If Social Media Dragons have control of your brain, it can make you feel worse about yourself and increase feelings of loneliness (social and spiritual circles). A growing number of studies have shown a connection between time spent on social media and feelings of anxiety and depression (psychological circle).[34]

When your brain is captive to Pornography Dragons, it may lead to instant gratification, but it doesn't lead to lasting satisfaction. In fact, it can reduce interest in real sex (psychological circle) and can come between you and your partner, leading to relationship troubles (social circle). It is also associated with increased risk of depression, anxiety, guilt, and anger (psychological circle).

## *How to Outfox the Digital Dragons*

1. **Recognize the Digital Dragons.** Understand that all of your devices, streaming services, news sites, social networks, and gaming and adult sites are Scheming Dragons.

2. **Look past the messenger.** Remember that major corporations are behind the games, movies, and gadgets you love. Remind yourself that the models enticing you to spend your time, attention, and money are only messengers. Corporations are cashing in on your use. TV anchors are usually attractive, friendly people who make you feel like you know them personally. You don't. You may think you're connecting with your friends on social media (beware: they may also be sharing news and fake news), but you're really giving your time and attention to the major corporation behind it.

3. **Get the whole picture before acting.** Ask yourself if your online activities are helping your brain or hurting it, building real relationships or hurting them. Are news sites reporting something that seems unbelievable or terribly frightening? Investigate. A few clicks can help you verify if a news story is factual. Ask yourself if you're spending time on social media because you're lonely and bored, and take stock if it's exacerbating some of your dragons.

4. **Don't make it easier for the Digital Dragons to hook you.** Don't sign up for alerts and notifications; turn off the "recommendations for you" feature if possible. Don't subscribe to adult sites. Don't follow news organizations on social media.

5. **Limit exposure to Digital Dragons.** Set time limits for your gadgets. Stick to the single-screen rule. Make your bedroom a technology-free zone. Take a tech time-out—even 15 minutes at a time can help. Set up blocks and filters on your devices. And don't watch or use any devices right before bedtime, or it may make it hard to sleep.

# CONTACT SPORTS DRAGONS

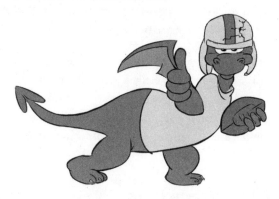

As mentioned earlier, your brain is soft and your skull is hard. Head injuries, even mild ones that occurred decades earlier, are a major cause of depression, addictions, and memory problems. A study from the Mayo Clinic found that one-third of people who played football at *any* level had lasting brain damage.[35] Oh no, I played football in high school, and it showed when I scanned myself decades later, but the good news was that my scan was much better after I implemented brain-healthy strategies.

The Super Bowl is one of the biggest events in the world. High-priced tickets for some boxing matches and mixed martial arts (MMA) bouts sell out in seconds. When there's a fight at an ice hockey match, that's what makes the evening news. The Scheming Dragons behind these contact sports are expert spin doctors who make head injuries seem like exciting entertainment. And they make billions of dollars each year at the expense of the health of millions of children, teenagers, and young adults who participate in these sports and try to emulate the hard hits, knockout punches, and scuffles they see on the sports highlights. The Contact Sports Dragons try to justify the injuries by touting the benefits that sports provide, such as physical exercise, teamwork, strategy, and lessons in overcoming adversity. These are all good, but you can easily get them in other sports that don't put you at risk of a head injury.

The NFL, the big daddy of Contact Sports Dragons, claims helmets make players safe, but this isn't true. According to an investigative article in *Sports Illustrated*, "Many of the assertions about helmet safety thrown around by today's manufacturers overstate the supporting science."[36] At Amen Clinics, we have been studying the association between football and brain injuries for several years. Our brain imaging work has shown clear evidence of traumatic brain injuries in kids and teens who play Pop Warner and high school football, in college players, and in current and retired NFL players. Our scans show that the more years they play football, the worse their brains look, and the damage starts early in the brain. This is why I have to admit that although most people lamented the loss of sports activities during the pandemic, I was actually very happy about the absence of contact sports.

*Contact Sports Dragons Consequences:* When your brain is always listening to the Contact Sports Dragons, you believe that playing football and other sports is "not that bad" and that head injuries won't cause lasting problems. This is a lie. Concussions, even ones that don't cause you to black out, can cause depression, anger, anxiety, memory loss, confusion, and more (biological and psychological circles).

### How to outfox the Contact Sports Dragons

1. **Recognize the Contact Sports Dragons.** Understand that schools, coaches, community sports programs, and parents can try to rope you into playing or promoting contact sports.

2. **Look past the messenger.** The professional athletes you see who are making millions of dollars are the exception. Most people who play sports never make any money from it, but they may be harmed for life by a head injury.

3. **Get the whole picture before acting.** Find out about the risk of concussions and head injuries before playing any sport.

4. **Don't make it easier for the Contact Sports Dragons to hook you.** If you want to send a message to these Scheming Dragons, don't watch their events on TV or pay for tickets to attend these sporting events.

5. **Limit exposure to Contact Sports Dragons.** Avoid playing or allowing your children to play contact sports. There are many alternatives, such as dance, tennis, table tennis, swimming, track, and golf.

If you've had a head injury, the good news is that many things can help it heal, even years later. Amen Clinics did the first and largest brain-imaging study on active and retired NFL players. The level of damage was alarming, but what really excited us was that on our program—which I call BRIGHT MINDS and which I wrote about in *Memory Rescue* and *The End of Mental Illness*—80 percent of our players showed significant improvement in blood flow, memory, attention, mood, and sleep.

# HOLIDAY DRAGONS

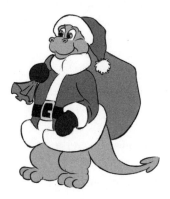

What could seem more festive and friendly than Holiday Dragons? These beasts promote holiday cheer and family togetherness, but they often end up causing stress, overspending, bad health, and suicidal thoughts. The Holiday Dragons put pressure on you to attend parties where you're encouraged to get in the spirit by overeating and drinking too much alcohol. There's nothing cheery about feeling bloated and hungover.

In our home, we refuse to feel deprived and make a conscious choice to eat healthy so we can feel energetic and happy and so we can celebrate the true meaning of the holidays. For example, at Thanksgiving, we want to stay focused on gratitude and being good role models for our family and the people we serve. Tana makes a brain-healthy meal that is so delicious some family members don't even realize they're eating nutrient-dense foods. Some of the dishes she's served for this holiday include marinated turkey (free-range, hormone-free, and antibiotic-free), "guiltless" gravy (with grass-fed butter or ghee, low-sodium chicken broth, arrowroot, coconut cream or milk, and flavorful herbs and spices), a cauliflower garlic mash (an amazing substitute for potatoes), a kale slaw (better than traditional coleslaw), and a yummy apple cinnamon crisp (with almond flour and a natural sugar alternative called erythritol). (Find these recipes on Tana's website at tanaamen. com/brain-healthy-thanksgiving-menu).

All those TV commercials and social-media posts showing families celebrating together can make you feel like you have to spend time with relatives you don't like or who are unhealthy to be around. You may not have one of those Hallmark families, you may not have any family at all, or you may have been unable to get together with loved ones during the pandemic, which can cause you to feel lonely and depressed.

Some of the most obnoxious Holiday Dragons are retailers who promote the spirit of giving, which translates into "buying" from them. More than 6 out of 10 people say they feel pressured to overspend during the holidays—whether it's on gifts, social occasions, travel, or charitable donations.[37]

The Holiday Dragons seem to always be with us:

New Year's Eve Dragons (party hats)
New Year's Day Dragons (floats)
Valentine's Day Dragons (cards, flowers, chocolates)
Super Bowl Dragons (team apparel)
St. Patrick's Day Dragons (green clothes and party favors)
Spring Break Dragons (swimsuits)
Easter Dragons (eggs, candy, new outfits)
Kentucky Derby Day Dragons (hats)
Cinco de Mayo Dragons (beer, tacos)
Mother's Day Dragons (flowers, cards)
Memorial Day Dragons (barbecues)
Father's Day Dragons (tools, cards)
Fourth of July Dragons (fireworks, patriotic apparel)
Labor Day Dragons (weekend getaways)
Halloween Dragons (costumes, candy, scary decorations)
Thanksgiving Dragons (too much food)
Christmas Eve Dragons (too much food)
Christmas Day Dragons (presents, too much food again)

*Holiday Dragons Consequences:* When your brain is always listening to the Holiday Dragons, you feel pressure to overeat, overspend, and overextend yourself. It can all lead to stress, loneliness, depression, anxiety (psychological circle), weight gain (biological circle), and trouble in your relationships (social circle).

### How to outfox the Holiday Dragons

1. **Recognize the Holiday Dragons.** Know that retailers are behind much of the pressure that comes with the holidays.

2. **Look past the messenger.** Santa Claus, the Easter Bunny, and Uncle Sam are cute and likable characters, but the real message is coming from those Scheming Holiday Dragons.

3. **Get the whole picture before acting.** Ask yourself if holiday-related activities are good for your brain or bad for your brain.

4. **Don't make it easier for the Holiday Dragons to hook you.** Don't sign up for notifications about sales and specials.

5. **Limit exposure to Holiday Dragons.** Make a plan for your holiday activities and spending. Let your family and friends know about your plans well ahead of time and ask for their support. Then stick to the plan.

## PROTECT OTHERS FROM THE SCHEMING DRAGONS

Learning to fight back against the Scheming Dragons in our society will help you ward off Bad Habit Dragons and damage to the four circles of health. The stronger your four circles are, the better you can identify and resist the Scheming Dragons. Protecting your loved ones from these beasts is equally important. Helping older parents and grandparents to identify and avoid the schemers who are trying to take advantage of them can keep them safe and secure. And teaching children from a young age to recognize schemers and to set boundaries will protect them from early harm and help them outfox the Scheming Dragons throughout their lifetime.

# ADDICTED DRAGON RECOVERY PROGRAM

## A NEW 12-STEP BRAIN-BASED MODEL

*Fairy tales are more than true: not because they tell us that dragons exist, but because they tell us that dragons can be beaten.*

NEIL GAIMAN, *CORALINE*

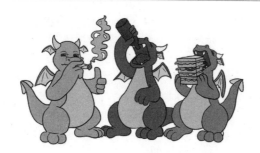

When Bad Habit and Scheming Dragons are left untamed for too long, or when your Dragon Tamer (PFC) is weak, you may become vulnerable to addictions. And high stress—such as a global pandemic that's threatening people's health, happiness, and livelihood—increases the susceptibility to addiction. The good news is that while plenty of people will abuse substances or engage in addictive behaviors and suffer consequences, they stop when they see the devastation their behavior causes. Yet a number of people will abuse substances or engage in self-destructive behaviors, have adverse consequences, and then continue their addictive choices despite the trouble. Take a look at some of my patients who have struggled with addictions.

Leslie, 23, had too much to drink at her company holiday party and came on to the boss . . . in front of his wife! She was fired the next day at work. Leslie felt humiliated and vowed never to get that drunk again. And she didn't.

Robbie, 25, went to his company's holiday party and got so trashed he went up to his supervisor and insulted her with a vulgar term in front of the company CEO. Robbie was fired on the spot. The next night, he went out to a bar with a friend to "celebrate" the fact that he didn't have to work with that "nasty woman" anymore. He got drunk again and was charged with a DUI as he drove home.

Derek, 16, was on the soccer team in high school. One day, he and his soccer teammates found a peephole to the girls' locker room where they saw the girls changing out of their clothes. A girl passing by outside noticed the group of guys, realized what they were doing, and turned them in to the school principal. Derek and his buddies got suspended for a week, and Derek never looked through a peephole again.

Brandon, 49, was only 14 years old when he peered through an open window to sneak a peek at his sister coming out of the shower. He felt an incredible rush, but his sister caught him in the act, told their parents, and got Brandon into big trouble. The next day, all Brandon could think about was the strong arousal he felt from watching her, so later that day, he peered through his sister's bedroom window to watch her change clothes. He got caught again, and his parents grounded him for a month. Years later, Brandon placed a hidden camera in the bathroom of an apartment he was renting out so he could watch his female tenant in the shower. She found the camera and sued Brandon for $1 million—even that didn't stop his voyeurism.

Tracy, 44, was so anxious about the coronavirus when safer-at-home orders were put in place that she went to the store and filled her cart with cupcakes, cheesecake, fudge brownies, and chocolate-covered pretzels. When she came home, she tore into the packages and stuffed them in her mouth. Within minutes of finishing her umpteen-thousand-calorie feast, she felt sick to her stomach. She spent most of the night throwing up, and the next day, she still felt queasy. She swore off bingeing and went back to her normal eating routine.

Stacey, 36, started bingeing 20 years ago when she got cut from the high school drill team. She went home and ate everything she could find in the kitchen cupboards. The sickness that followed didn't deter her from doing it again when her boyfriend dumped her, when she didn't get into her first-choice college, or when she didn't land the job she wanted. Even the fact that she had gained 30 pounds and hated the way she looked couldn't keep her from bingeing whenever something bad or stressful happened in her life.

What's the difference between those who overdo it with alcohol, food, sex, or other addictive behaviors but learn from their mistakes and those who minimize the consequences and continue in the same destructive behaviors over and over? For the latter group, an army of Dragons from the Past; They, Them, and Other Dragons; Bad Habit Dragons; and Scheming Dragons, along with a weak Dragon Tamer, overwhelm them to such a degree that Addicted Dragons kidnap their brains and their lives.

Slaying Addicted Dragons is complicated, and it requires more than an alert and healthy PFC (see section 7 for more on the Dragon Tamer). It requires addressing all four circles of health—biological, psychological, social, and spiritual—taming other dragons, and healing your brain.

## A LOOK AT 12-STEP PROGRAMS

Let me start by writing that I'm a fan of Alcoholics Anonymous and other 12-step programs. I have seen AA, along with Narcotics Anonymous (NA), Cocaine Anonymous (CA), Overeaters Anonymous (OA), and similar programs change people's lives, including the life of my own family members. I have referred patients to them for decades. Yet when AA was started in 1935, the founders did not have access to sophisticated neuroimaging techniques, and they never considered the brain as an integral part of treatment, unaware of the biological circle of health. The 12 steps of the anonymous programs often do address psychological, social, and spiritual steps.

P **Step 1:** We admitted we were powerless over alcohol—that our lives had become unmanageable.

SP **Step 2:** Came to believe that a power greater than ourselves could restore us to sanity. (There is hope for healing.)

SP **Step 3:** Made a decision to turn our will and our lives over to the care of God as we understood Him. (Ask for help and trust the process.)

(P) **Step 4:** Made a searching and fearless moral inventory of ourselves. (Acknowledge our faults and the effect our behavior is having on others.)

(S) (SP) **Step 5:** Admitted to God, ourselves, and to another human being the exact nature of our wrongs. (Confession is helpful to alleviate guilt and shame.)

(SP) **Step 6:** Were entirely ready to have God remove all these defects of character. (Let go of the behaviors holding you back.)

(P) (SP) **Step 7:** Humbly asked Him to remove our shortcomings. (Admit when we are wrong and ask for help to be better.)

(P) (S) **Step 8:** Made a list of all persons we had harmed and became willing to make amends to them all. (Prepare to apologize and make amends to those we hurt.)

(S) **Step 9:** Made direct amends to such people wherever possible, except when to do so would injure them or others. (Be thoughtful in how you apologize and make amends.)

(P) **Step 10:** Continued to take personal inventory and when we were wrong promptly admitted it. (Never end your improvement.)

(S) **Step 11:** Sought through prayer and meditation to improve our conscious contact with God as we understood Him, praying only for knowledge of His will for us and the power to carry that out. (Stay connected to a new way of living.)

(S) (SP) **Step 12:** Having had a spiritual awakening as the result of these steps, we tried to carry this message [of AA, CA, NA, OA, etc.] and to practice these principles in all our affairs. (Help others.)[1]

Anonymous programs are powerful, time-tested, and have worked for millions of people around the world. Yet they clearly do not work for everyone. A study conducted by the Department of Veterans Affairs showed 43 percent of attendees were sober at 18 months.[2] One of the reasons for the lower efficacy is that this program and many other recovery programs include no steps to address the physical functioning of the brain, which is the missing link to breaking any addiction. With this in mind, let me offer 12 new steps to breaking the chains of addiction and help your Addicted Dragons stay in recovery. I'll use a more balanced biological, psychological, social, and spiritual model, as all four of these circles are important.

# 12 NEW STEPS TO HEAL YOUR ADDICTED DRAGONS

*Step 1: Know what you want.*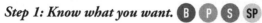

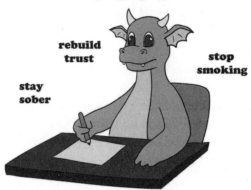

Most addiction-recovery programs start with acknowledging trouble, by knowing when you are powerless over a substance or behavior. I think we should start one step earlier by knowing exactly what you want in life. If you tell your brain what you want, it can help make it happen.

In the addiction world, therapists will often ask clients if they have a *high bottom* (you learn quickly) or a *low bottom* (you have to lose everything before you get help). When I was 16, I got drunk on a six-pack of Michelob and a half bottle of champagne. I was sick for three days and have had very little alcohol since then. I often wonder why other people think it's fun. For me, it wasn't, plus I acted like a fool, which was embarrassing. So I have a high bottom. Actor Chris Browning, star of *Bosch*, *Westworld*, and *Sons of Anarchy*, joined us in 2020 on our podcast, *The Brain Warrior's Way*. He told my wife, Tana, and me that he used heroin for six years. He went from having a beachfront home in Malibu to being homeless under the 405 freeway and was arrested multiple times before he finally got sober. He has a low bottom. Some people are more motivated to avoid pain (me), while others are motivated by pleasure (Chris). Which are you? Do you learn from mistakes early or late? No one starts out wanting to have a low bottom. But addiction makes it easy to lose sight of what's most important to you.

My friend Dr. David Smith, founder of the famous Haight Ashbury Free Clinic in San Francisco, told me a story about attending a medical conference in Chicago in 1989 when he got a frantic call from Bill Graham, the legendary rock concert promoter. Graham was on tour with the Grateful Dead and told David, "Jerry Garcia is strung out, and you have to do something." David headed to the band's hotel, where he had to snake his way through a sea of tie-dye-clad groupies and billows of marijuana smoke to get to Garcia's room.

Inside, he was welcomed by Graham and Garcia's bandmates: bass player, Phil Lesh, and rhythm guitarist, Bob Weir, who was in recovery from hard drugs.

Drugs and rock and roll had been a way of life for Garcia for decades. While on tour with the Dead, people would give him all the drugs he wanted. He would often smoke heroin backstage just to make himself feel better. The years of hard partying and touring had not been kind to Garcia. He was severely overweight, had diabetes, and had even slipped into a diabetic coma a few years earlier. But that wasn't enough to make him want to change his ways.

The band told Garcia that he was killing himself with drugs, and they were staging an intervention. It wasn't the first intervention they had tried. Garcia had run away from the last one and subsequently gotten arrested for possession. This time, though, his bandmates told him that they would no longer go out on the road with him unless he got help for his addiction. For Garcia, touring with the band and playing music for thousands of people was what he loved most in life. The threat of losing that is what finally motivated him to change and enter a holistic addiction treatment center.

In order for you to break free from the chains of addiction, you must know what you want in life. What do you want in your relationships, work, money, and physical, emotional, and spiritual health? Write it down in the One Page Miracle exercise on page 259. Then ask yourself every day, *Is my behavior getting me what I want?* Does your behavior serve your goals or hurt them? Does it fit? If not, it's time to work a program.

---

*If you don't make a conscious effort to visualize who you are and what you want in life, then you empower other people and circumstances [including addictions] to shape you and your life by default.*[3]

STEPHEN COVEY

---

*Step 2: Know when your Addicted Dragons have taken you hostage.*

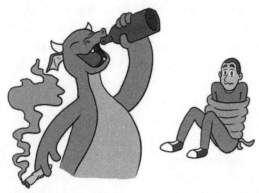

This step is similar to Step 1 in the AA model. Know when you are powerless and your life is unmanageable. So how do you know when you are in trouble? Many people are in denial about their behavior and are very slow to admit when they have a problem. I often tell my patients the answer is simple: You're an addict when your behavior (drinking, drugs, eating, shopping, gambling, sex, etc.) gets you into trouble with your relationships, health, work, money, or the law—and you do it again. You don't learn that the behavior gets you into trouble, or you cannot stop it.

For many people, problem behaviors creep up slowly, and the changes are hard to notice. By the time you are in the grasp of the Addicted Dragons, your brain has rewired itself and it drives you to continue the addiction in spite of consequences. Take the quiz on page 204 to find out if you might have a problem. It is called the CAGE Assessment and addiction experts have used it for decades to help identify drinking problems. These same questions can also help you pinpoint problems with other substances and behaviors. Simply substitute the word *drinking* with *smoking, prescription drug use, overeating, internet porn viewing, shopping, gambling,* or whatever your addiction may be.

### SIGNS YOU MAY HAVE A PROBLEM

Addicted Dragons can impact every aspect of your life, including your physical, mental, and emotional health; social life; and core values. They also fuel other dragons. The problems can be biological, psychological, social, or spiritual. Most people with a problem will exhibit issues in several, if not all, of these areas. Here is an example:

Cole was a shy, quiet 16-year-old who loved playing the piano and being in the math club. When one of his older brother's friends introduced him to cocaine, he immediately loved the way it melted away his shyness and made him feel more outgoing, talkative, and energetic. When he used it, his friends

202 * **YOUR BRAIN IS ALWAYS LISTENING**

said he was the life of the party, and girls seemed to like him more. So he started using it whenever he went to a party. Then he began snorting a few lines before school events, and then he did it every morning before he got to school. He rarely felt hungry anymore and lost about 15 pounds, leaving him rail thin.

When Cole was high, he talked a mile a minute and fidgeted in his seat in class. But when the effects wore off, he went back to his old introverted self, felt depressed, and could barely muster the energy to get off the couch. He quit taking piano lessons, dropped out of the math club, and dumped his old friends in order to spend more time with his new drug buddies. When he couldn't get his hands on any cocaine, he couldn't stop thinking about it and lashed out at his parents and younger sister whenever they asked him if he was using drugs. Cole was in the clutches of his Addicted Dragons.

*Biological Symptoms*
Biological signs include changes to physical health and appearance and include, but are not limited to, the following:

- Increase in cravings for the substance or behavior
- Changes in eating or sleeping habits
- Feeling sick or hung over
- Forgetting what happened while under the influence
- Using increasing amounts of a substance to get the same feeling
- Inability to quit without feeling physically ill

*Psychological Symptoms*
Addictions also result in many psychological issues:

- Depression, irritability, or mood swings
- Loss of interest in favorite activities
- Minimizing the consequences of behavior
- Annoyance or irritation when others question you
- Feelings of guilt about behavior
- Feeling anxious, depressed, or irritable when you are unable to engage in the behavior
- Spending the day thinking about the behavior
- Feeling powerless to change your behavior

*Social Symptoms*
Harmful behaviors can cause many problems in your social life:

- Negative changes in work or school performance
- Withdrawal from family and friends
- Neglecting responsibilities
- Becoming friends with people who share your addiction
- Spending more and more time engaging in the behavior
- Avoiding situations where you can't engage in the behavior
- Befriending the wrong people who are more likely to engage in harmful behavior

*Spiritual Symptoms*
In this context, *spiritual* doesn't mean "religious." It refers to your core values and morals, which are typically compromised in people with addictions and other troublesome behaviors. For example, before you became a slave to your habit, you probably never would have lied to your spouse, stolen money from a friend, or forgotten to pick up the kids from school. When you become entangled in problem behaviors, however, you start to do things you used to think were wrong. The following are a few symptoms of a broken moral compass:

- Breaking rules at home, at school, or in the community
- Cheating
- Lying to family, friends, significant others, coworkers, and others
- Stealing or selling cherished personal items to fuel your addiction
- Hiding things
- Breaking promises and making excuses
- Using language only people with your addiction would understand

As you look at these lists of symptoms, be honest with yourself about the changes in your behavior and life. Take a pen and circle the symptoms that sound like you. The more symptoms you circle, the more likely there is a problem. Unless you recognize and admit that you have a problem, you will not be able to get your Addicted Dragons into recovery.

# CAGE ASSESSMENT*

HAVE YOU EVER FELT YOU SHOULD **C**UT DOWN ON YOUR DRINKING (OR OTHER BEHAVIOR)?

- ○ YES
- ○ NO

HAVE PEOPLE **A**NNOYED YOU BY CRITICIZING YOUR DRINKING (OR OTHER BEHAVIOR)?

- ○ YES
- ○ NO

HAVE YOU EVER FELT BAD OR **G**UILTY ABOUT YOUR DRINKING (OR OTHER BEHAVIOR)?

- ○ YES
- ○ NO

HAVE YOU EVER HAD A DRINK (OR ENGAGED IN OTHER BEHAVIOR) FIRST THING IN THE MORNING (AS AN "**E**YE OPENER") TO STEADY YOUR NERVES OR GET RID OF A HANGOVER?

- ○ YES
- ○ NO

IF YOU ANSWERED YES TO TWO OR MORE OF THESE QUESTIONS, THEN YOU MAY HAVE A PROBLEM.

---

*John A. Ewing, "Detecting Alcoholism: The CAGE Questionnaire," *Journal of the American Medical Association* 252, no. 14 (October 12, 1984): 1905–07.

*Step 3: Make a decision to care for, balance, and repair your brain.* **B**

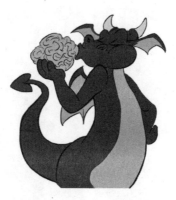

The missing link in nearly all addiction-treatment programs worldwide is that very few of them look at and assess brain function on a routine basis. Your brain is involved in everything you do and everything you are. When your brain works right, you work right, but when it is troubled for any reason, you are much more likely to have trouble in your life, especially with Addicted Dragons. You can diligently work all the anonymous steps (AA, NA, CA, etc.) with energy, enthusiasm, and commitment, but if your brain is not working at an optimal level (and most brains aren't), you will have a much harder time getting and staying sober, despite your best efforts.

When I first started looking at the brain in 1991, it revolutionized my thinking and clinical practice. At the time, I was the director of an in-patient substance abuse treatment program, and the SPECT scans of my addicted patients were terrible compared to my other patients with psychiatric issues, such as anxiety, depression, or ADHD. It was clear that drugs and alcohol damaged brains; and if they damaged brains, they were damaging lives. Over time, it also became clear that pornography, gambling addictions, and video-game addictions also damaged brains.

**HEALTHY SURFACE SPECT SCAN**

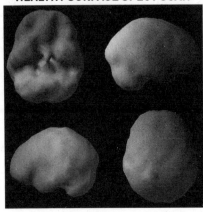

**ALCOHOL-DAMAGED SURFACE SPECT SCAN**

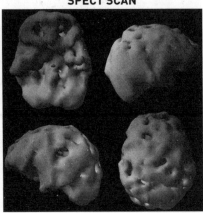

**COCAINE-DAMAGED SURFACE SPECT SCAN**

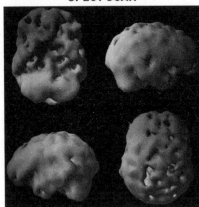

**INHALANT-DAMAGED SURFACE SPECT SCAN**

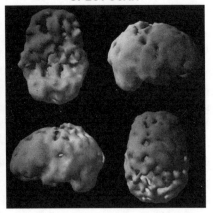

To beat any addiction, it is critical to understand and optimize the brain. You must fall in love with it, and work to balance and repair it, so it can control all of the dragons (Dragons of the Past; They, Them, and Other Dragons; Bad Habit Dragons; Scheming Dragons) and ANTs that steal your happiness. Eating right, exercising, avoiding anything that hurts your brain, and engaging in regular brain-healthy habits are critical to beating any addiction. However, at addiction-support groups, you're likely to see people smoking, drinking coffee, and offering one another unhealthy snacks.

I once helped a well-known addiction-treatment center in Florida add brain SPECT imaging to their evaluation services. I was excited about the expansion of my work until I saw what they were feeding their clients for breakfast the morning of my first lecture: doughnuts, pastries, fruit juices, and sugary cereals. Sugar is another addictive substance. This must change. If you want to beat addictions, it is critical you get your brain right—and the food right. In my book *The End of Mental Illness*, I include an entire chapter on simple brain-healthy rules that make food insanely simple. For dozens of brain-healthy recipes, visit our site at mybrainfitlife.com.

*Step 4. Reach for forgiveness for yourself and others.* **B** **P** **S** **SP**

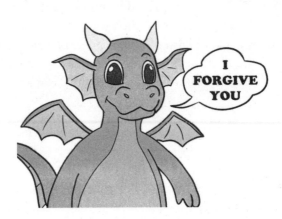

The easy answer for addictions is that people should just stop the difficult behavior. Their Addicted Dragons should just go to sleep and stop bothering everyone. Addiction is much more complicated than most people think. Our brain-imaging work taught me that tough love works for people whose brains work right; but for people with troubled brains, tough love is like doing software programming on people with hardware problems, which is not very effective.

Critical to beating any addiction are self-love, self-care, and forgiveness of yourself and others. If you do not love yourself, you won't take proper care of your brain, and you will likely continue to hurt it. Forgiveness is the gift that keeps on giving; it is powerful medicine. Research shows a connection between forgiveness and reduced anxiety, depression, and psychiatric disorders. It is also associated with having fewer physical health symptoms and a lower mortality rate.[4] See page 53 in section 1 for the REACH model of forgiveness (also the key to defeating the Judgmental Dragons).

## Step 5: Know your Addicted Dragon's brain type. B

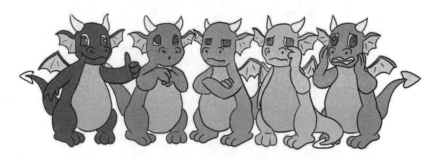

All brains, even healthy ones, are not the same. When we first started to do brain-imaging work at the Amen Clinics, we were looking for patterns associated with certain illnesses. We discovered they all have multiple patterns that require their own unique treatments. That made sense because, for example, there will never be just one pattern for depression because not all depressed people are the same. Some are withdrawn, others are angry, and still others are anxious or obsessive. Taking a one-size-fits-all approach invites failure and frustration.

The scans also helped us discover different brain types, which created nuances to patients' problems and treatments. This one idea led to a dramatic breakthrough in our effectiveness with patients, and it opened up a new world of understanding and hope for the tens of thousands of people who have come to see us and the millions of people who have read my books or seen my shows. Understanding these brain types is critical to getting the right help. Here is a summary of five basic brain types and the treatments for each one.[5] You may have more than one brain type as there are 16 possible combinations.

### BRAIN TYPE 1: BALANCED

People with this type tend to have healthy brains overall and be focused, flexible, positive, and relaxed. Their brains tend to be healthy, which makes them less likely to have Addicted Dragons. However, it's important for these people to love and care for their brain with general brain-healthy strategies, such as regular exercise, a balanced diet, and ongoing new learning. These people benefit from taking a multiple vitamin/mineral supplement and omega-3 fatty acids and from testing and optimizing their vitamin D levels. Not caring about their brain, being bad to their brain, or putting their brain at risk (by playing tackle football, for example) can increase their vulnerability to Addicted Dragons.

## HEALTHY BRAIN SURFACE SPECT SCAN

Full, even, symmetrical activity

**BRAIN TYPE 2: SPONTANEOUS**
People with this brain type tend to be:

- Spontaneous
- Risk-taking
- Creative, out-of-the-box thinkers
- Restless
- Easily distracted
- Focused only when interested

The SPECT scans of this type typically have lower activity in the front of the brain in the PFC. So their Dragon Tamer is often weak. The PFC stops us from saying or doing things that are not in our best interest, but it can also stop creative, out-of-the-box thinking. The Spontaneous brain type tends to be associated with lower dopamine levels in the brain and may cause people to be more restless and risk-taking, and to struggle to stay focused on something unless their interest in it is high. Our research team has published several studies showing that when people with this brain type try to concentrate, they actually have less activity in the PFC, which causes them to need excitement or stimulation in order to focus (think of firefighters and race-car drivers). Smokers and heavy coffee drinkers also tend to fit this type of brain, as they use these substances to turn their brains "on."

Take Randall, for example. He started smoking when he was 16 years old, and at age 51, he decided to quit. Every morning, he woke up with good intentions, but the moment he saw someone else smoking, he would impulsively reach for his cigarettes. Randall came to see us for other issues, and his SPECT scans showed low PFC activity. With the following strategies to boost activity in the PFC naturally, he was finally able to stick with a program to quit smoking.

### SPONTANEOUS BRAIN TYPE

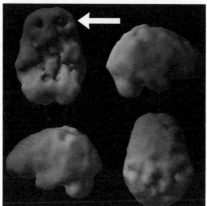

Low prefrontal cortex activity at front of brain

Any supplement or medicine that calms the brain, such as 5-hydroxytryptophan (5-HTP) or selective serotonin reuptake inhibitors (SSRIs), may make the Spontaneous brain type worse, as it will lower the already low PFC function, which can then take the brakes off the person's behavior. We have treated many people who had done things they later regretted, such as becoming hypersexual or spending money they did not have, when they started taking SSRIs. It turned out they had low activity in the PFC, and the serotonin-boosting medications diminished their judgment.

This brain type is optimized by increasing dopamine levels to strengthen the PFC. Higher-protein, lower-carbohydrate diets tend to help, as do physical exercise and certain stimulating supplements, such as rhodiola, green tea extract, L-theanine, ashwagandha, panax ginseng, ginkgo biloba, and phosphatidylserine. Try them in the order listed here for a few days each to see which work best for you. If one or more overstimulates or upsets you, stop taking it and move on to the next in the list.

☐ *Rhodiola,* an herb grown at high altitudes in Asia and Europe, has been traditionally used to fight fatigue, improve memory, and increase attention span. Look for Rhodiola rosea root standardized to contain 3 percent rosavins and a minimum of one percent salidrosides. The typical adult dose is 170–200 mg twice a day.

☐ *Green tea leaf extract* is made from the dried leaves of *Camellia sinensis*, an evergreen shrub. It has been used to improve focus and as a remedy for many ailments, including anxiety and weight loss. The typical dose is 200–300 mg.

☐ *L-theanine* is an amino acid uniquely found in green tea. It can increase dopamine. It also increases GABA and serotonin, so it tends to have a balancing effect on the brain. It helps with focus as well as mental and physical stress. The typical dose is 100–200 mg two to three times a day.

☐ *Ashwagandha* (*Withania somnifera*, Indian ginseng, Indian Winter Cherry) is commonly used to help with focus and relaxation. The plant itself is an adaptogen, with properties that enable the body to better handle stress, anxiety, and fatigue. The recommended dose is 125 mg twice a day.

☐ *Phosphatidylserine* (PS) is essential to brain health as it maintains neurons and neuronal networks so that the brain can continue to form and retain memories. Positron emission tomography (PET) studies, similar to SPECT, of patients who have taken PS show that it produces a general increase in metabolic activity in the brain.[6] The typical adult dose is 100–300 mg a day.

### BRAIN TYPE 3: PERSISTENT

People with this brain type tend to:

- Be persistent
- Be relentless or strong-willed
- Like things a certain way
- Get "stuck" on thoughts
- Hold on to hurts
- See what is wrong in themselves or others

Take-charge people who won't take no for an answer are likely to have this brain type. The Persistent brain type often has increased activity in the front part of the brain, in the anterior cingulate gyrus (ACG)—what I have described previously as the brain's gear shifter. It helps people go from thought to thought or move from action to action and is involved with being mentally flexible and going with the flow. They tend to be tenacious and stubborn. In addition, they may worry, have trouble sleeping, be argumentative and oppositional, and hold grudges from the past. When the ACG is overactive, usually due to low levels of serotonin, people can have problems shifting attention, which can make them persist—even when it may not be a good idea for them to do so.

For instance, Leigh, 42, couldn't stop thinking about gambling. The minute he woke up, he powered up his computer to check the spread on the day's sporting events. On a single game, he would often bet not only on which team would win, but also on half-time scores, individual player stats, and more. He came to our clinics because his wife was threatening to divorce him if he didn't stop gambling and because he worried incessantly and held grudges. His brain SPECT study showed too much activity in the ACG. Taking natural supplements to boost serotonin helped him overcome his constant worrying. Combined with psychotherapy and attendance at a gambling support group, he was finally able to tame his Addicted Dragons.

Caffeine and diet pills tend to make this brain type worse because it does not need more stimulation. Indeed, people who have a Persistent brain type may feel as though they need a glass of wine, or two or three, at night to calm their worries.

**HEALTHY ACTIVE SPECT SCAN**    **PERSISTENT BRAIN TYPE**

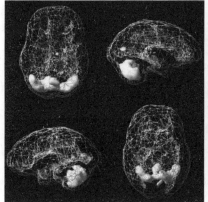
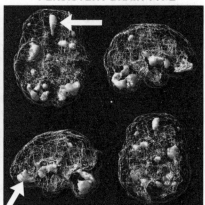

Most active areas in cerebellum
at back of brain

High anterior cingulate
activity at front of brain

High-glycemic carbohydrates like bread, pasta, and sweets turn to sugar quickly and increase serotonin, which is calming to the brain. That's why Persistent brain types can become addicted to these simple carbohydrates. They often use carbs as "mood foods" to self-medicate an underlying mood issue. It is best to avoid these quick fixes because they can cause long-term health problems. Instead, use physical exercise to boost serotonin and consider taking supplements, such as 5-hydroxytryptophan (5-HTP) and saffron.

☐ *5-hydroxytryptophan*, or *5-HTP*, is an amino acid precursor (this means it is converted) to serotonin. 5-HTP boosts serotonin levels in the brain and helps to calm ACG hyperactivity (greasing the cingulate, if you will, to improve shifting one's attention). A number of double-blind studies have shown that it is also an effective mood enhancer[7] and appetite suppressor.[8] The recommended adult dose of 5-HTP is 50–200 mg a day.

☐ *Saffron*, one of the world's most expensive spices, has seen a research boom showing it is helpful for mood,[9] memory,[10] and sexuality.[11] The recommended adult dosage is 15 mg twice a day.

**BRAIN TYPE 4: SENSITIVE**
People with this brain type tend to:

- Be sensitive
- Feel deeply
- Be empathic
- Struggle with moods
- Be more pessimistic
- Struggle with negative thoughts

The SPECT scans of the Sensitive brain type generally show increased activity in the limbic or emotional centers of the brain, making these people sensitive, empathic, and deeply feeling but also subject to issues with their moods. They may also struggle with being more pessimistic and having negative thoughts.

As a freshman in college, Danielle started having persistent feelings of despair and sadness that she couldn't shake. While home for the holidays, she found some OxyContin left over from her dad's root canal surgery and decided to try one. The drug made her feel happy and truly alive. She took the rest of the pills back to college, and when they were gone, she started buying them from a guy at school. When her regular supplier disappeared, she bought it from a new guy who turned out to be an undercover cop. Danielle got arrested and wound up in court-ordered drug treatment and eventually came to see us for a scan. Her SPECT scan showed increased activity in the deep limbic system. With a combination of an addiction-treatment program, natural supplements (see below), and brain-healthy lifestyle changes, Danielle was able to fight off her Addicted Dragons to regain control of her life and her happiness.

| HEALTHY ACTIVE SPECT SCAN | SENSITIVE BRAIN TYPE |
|---|---|
| 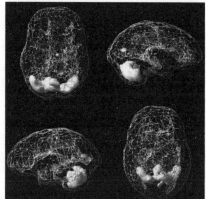 | 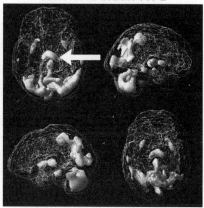 |
| Most active areas in cerebellum at back of brain | High deep limbic activity (arrow) |

Exercise and specific supplements may help the Sensitive brain type. If someone with this type is also a Persistent brain type (yes, it's possible to be a combination of types), the supplements or medications that boost serotonin may help the most.

☐ *S-adenosyl-methionine*, or *SAMe*, is crucial for the production of several neurotransmitters (dopamine, epinephrine, and serotonin).[12] Taking SAMe has been shown to have antidepressant qualities.[13] A 2017 comprehensive review by the American Psychiatric Association Council on Research Work Group found SAMe clearly effective against depression. SAMe has also been found to reduce joint inflammation and pain. People who have a tendency toward bipolar disorder should check with their doctor before trying this supplement. The typical adult dose is 400–800 mg twice a day. Usually, it is best taken early in the day as it may be more stimulating for some.

☐ *Omega-3 fatty acids* are important for healthy moods. Low levels of these fatty acids have been linked to depression, suicidal behavior, and many other biological and psychological issues. At Amen Clinics in 2016 we tested the omega-3 fatty acid levels of 50 consecutive patients who were not taking fish oil supplements. We found that 49 out of 50 had suboptimal levels. In a separate study on 130 patients, cognitive testing showed that low levels of omega-3 were associated with lower scores in mood.[14] The typical adult dose is 1,000–2,000 mg a day.

☐ *Vitamin D* is essential for brain health, stable moods, memory, and many other bodily processes. We test the vitamin D levels of all our patients at Amen Clinics, and a staggering percentage are low in this important vitamin. The lower your vitamin D levels, the more likely you are to suffer from the blues. Decades of research point to an association between low levels of vitamin D and mood problems, such as depression. Supplementation may help, according to a 2008 study in the *Journal of Internal Medicine* that followed 441 overweight and obese adults with depression for one year.[15] In this study, individuals who took vitamin D (20,000 IU or 40,000 IU per week) reported a significant decrease in their depressive symptoms, but those who took a placebo did not see such improvement. The dose suggestion is 2,000 IUs a day or more, depending on your level. (Have your health-care provider check your level with a blood test called 25-hydroxyvitamin D.)

### BRAIN TYPE 5: CAUTIOUS

People with this brain type tend to be:

- Prepared
- Cautious
- Motivated
- Reserved
- Busy-minded
- Restless

On SPECT images, we often see heightened activity in the anxiety centers of the brain, such as the basal ganglia, insular cortex, or amygdala. The neurotransmitter GABA helps calm overfiring in the brain, and low levels of GABA frequently cause people with this brain type to struggle more with anxiety and subsequently be more cautious and reserved. However, on the flip side, they also tend to be more prepared.

Amanda, 25, felt nervous all the time and would stop at the bar on her way home from her high-stress job in advertising to unwind with a few drinks. Even though she drank every day, she never felt drunk or out of control, so she didn't think she was addicted. When she came to our clinics at the urging of her boyfriend, we found that her brain had a toxic appearance, indicating damage from the alcohol. Her brain also showed too much activity in the basal ganglia. With a treatment plan that included relaxation techniques, combined with natural supplements (see below), she felt calmer and was able to stop relying on alcohol to soothe her nerves.

**HEALTHY ACTIVE SPECT SCAN**

**CAUTIOUS BRAIN TYPE**

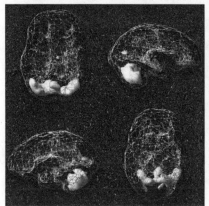

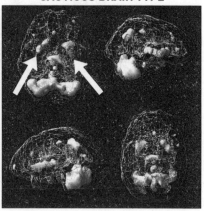

Most active areas in cerebellum
at back of brain

High basal ganglia activity (arrow)

Prayer, meditation, and hypnosis can help soothe this brain type, as can a combination of vitamin B6 (25 mg), magnesium glycinate, malate or citrate (the forms of magnesium that have optimum bioavailability; take 150–300 mg two to three times a day), and GABA, the calming neurotransmitter (250–750 mg two to three times a day).

It is common to have more than one brain type; all of the potential combinations add up to sixteen types, such as Spontaneous-Persistent-Sensitive or Sensitive-Cautious. Many years ago, we realized that not everyone can come to one of our clinics to get scanned, so based on thousands of scans, we've developed a questionnaire that helps predict what your brain might look like. The questionnaire is not as good as actually looking at the brain, but it is still helpful and used by thousands of medical and mental health professionals around the world. Find out your brain type as part of our free Brain Health Assessment at brainhealthassessment.com, where we also have specific suggestions to help each type.

*Step 6: Lock up the Craving Dragons.* 🅑 🅟

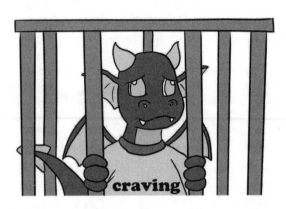

All of us are vulnerable to cravings, but when you also have Addicted Dragons, just seeing a glass pipe used for smoking cocaine, smelling cookies baking at the food court at the mall, or seeing an ad for a new video game will spark the emotional memory centers in your brain and trigger cravings to indulge in your old behavior. Even after decades of sobriety or steering clear of gambling, bulimia, video games, or porn, your brain is still vulnerable to cravings and those old patterns of behavior.

One of my patients, Molly, knew her risk. At 58, she had to have a surgical procedure. She was 32 years clean from a heroin addiction. When her doctor prescribed Vicodin—an opiate like heroin—for post-surgical pain relief, just taking one fired up the old addicted pathway in her brain and ratcheted up cravings for the drug she had quit so many years before. Fortunately, Molly had anticipated this could be a problem, and she had given the bottle of Vicodin to her husband and put him in charge of hiding them from her, counting them out each day, and dispensing them to her as directed on the bottle. After a couple of days, her pain was more bearable, and she switched to nonopiate, over-the-counter pain relievers, and the cravings subsided.

It is critical to learn how to keep cravings at bay. The following nine strategies will help you get control of your cravings so you can avoid relapse.

1. **Keep your blood sugar balanced.** Low blood-sugar levels are associated with lower overall brain activity, including lower activity in the PFC, the Dragon Tamer. Low brain activity here means more cravings, bad decisions, and relapse. Low blood-sugar levels can make you feel hungry, irritable, or anxious—all of which make you more likely to make poor choices. Low blood-sugar levels can also fuel anger and increase distractibility.

What causes low blood-sugar levels? Many everyday behaviors can cause dips in blood-sugar levels, including drinking alcohol, skipping meals, and consuming sugary snacks or beverages. High-sugar treats and drinks cause an initial spike in blood sugar but then a crash about 30 minutes later. Plus, the body uses glucose less efficiently as the day progresses, leading to more self-control failures in the evening and later at night. Keep your blood-sugar levels even throughout the day so you can reduce cravings and boost your self-control.

*Eat a nutritious breakfast every day.* Eating a nutrient-rich breakfast, including protein, helps your blood sugar get off to a good start and can keep it balanced for hours so you don't get hungry before lunchtime.

*Have smaller meals throughout the day.* This helps eliminate the blood-sugar roller coaster that can impact your emotions and increase your cravings.

*Stay away from simple sugars and refined carbohydrates.* This includes candy, sodas, cookies, crackers, white rice, white bread, and sweetened fruit juices. Foods that are high in sugar and fat work on the addiction centers of your brain. This is critical not only for people who are addicted to overeating, but also for people with other addictions. Bingeing on sugar has been found to alter brain chemistry and raise the risk for indulging in other drugs or alcohol. Sugar addiction is common in alcoholics and often develops when alcoholics try to quit drinking. Because the body metabolizes alcohol the same way as sugar, eating sugar can fuel alcohol cravings, and vice versa.

*Avoid the dessert table.* When I got this one idea through my own thick skull, I was finally able to lose the extra pounds I had been trying to shed for years. I love living without cravings. But for years, I fought the idea of giving up sweets, like Rocky Road ice cream or candy. I thought the key to losing weight was simply about calories in versus calories out. If I stayed within a certain calorie range, I'd be fine. The problem was that eating the sugar activated my cravings and made it very hard to stay away from foods that were bad for me.

For most people, it takes about two weeks of completely avoiding sugar for your dessert cravings to go away.

2. **Decrease the artificial sweeteners.** If you really want to decrease your cravings, you also have to get rid of the artificial sweeteners in your diet. We think of these sweeteners as free because they have no calories, but because they are up to 600 times sweeter than sugar, they may activate the appetite centers of the brain, making you crave even more food and more sugar. A group of Australian scientists found that alcohol floods the bloodstream faster when it is mixed with beverages containing artificial sweeteners rather than sugar. Diet sodas are not the answer. The "natural" no-calorie sweeteners I like are stevia, erythritol, and xylitol because they don't impact blood-sugar levels. However, I still recommend them only as an occasional treat.

3. **Manage your stress.** Another important way to decrease your cravings is to get on a daily stress-management program. Anything stressful can trigger certain hormones that activate your cravings, making you believe that you need the ice cream, cigarettes, or cocaine, or that you must take a virtual break, kick something to blow off steam, or call a friend to complain about your day. Prayer, meditation, and hypnosis are wonderful stress-management practices that can help boost your brain to control your cravings.

4. **Outsmart sneaky addiction triggers.** If you're an overeater, you can't go to the mall, airport, or ball game without seeing store after store and vendor after vendor advertising something that will fire up your cravings. For example, whenever I went to the movies, I used to immediately think about getting a big tub of popcorn with lots of butter along with licorice. But then I actually thought about the gobs of saturated fat, salt, and sugar that would be flooding my brain.

   To control your cravings, you have to know the people, places, and things that fuel your cravings so you can plan ahead for vulnerable times. For example, I take a snack with me when I go to the movies now so I am not tempted by the popcorn and licorice.

5. **Find out about hidden food allergies.** Hidden food allergies and food sensitivities can trigger cravings and make you relapse. For example, did you know that wheat gluten and milk allergies can

decrease blood flow to the brain and decrease your judgment? In addition, many of the symptoms associated with food allergies, such as headaches, sleep problems, lack of concentration, anger, aggression, and anxiety, can increase stress and cravings along with other harmful behaviors.

Food allergies are closely linked to alcoholism. Corn, wheat, rye, and barley are common sources of food allergies and happen to be ingredients used to make alcohol like vodka, whiskey, beer, gin, and bourbon. The foods that you are allergic to are often the ones you crave the most, so if you are allergic to an ingredient in alcohol, you may crave alcohol.

6. **Train willpower.** Willpower is like a muscle. You have to use it or lose it. Most of us learn to develop self-control as children. When our parents say no to us when we ask if we can do something that isn't good for us—have a plate of cookies before dinner, ride on the back of a neighbor's motorcycle without a helmet, or grab the tail of a strange dog—we learn to say no to ourselves. But maybe your parents weren't around much because they were workaholics and you had free rein to do whatever you wanted so you never learned self-control. Or perhaps your parents had addictions, and you learned to give in to your desires by watching their behavior. Maybe your Addicted Dragons have robbed you of your ability to say no. Or perhaps your Bad Habit Dragons have trained your brain to give in to your cravings.

No matter what the reason is for your lack of self-restraint, pump up your willpower by practicing it. Say no to the things that are not good for you over and over. The more you do this, the easier it will be. Once you've said no, immediately do something else to move your focus off your craving. Redirect your attention.

7. **Get moving.** Scientific research on exercise and addiction has found that physical activity can cut cravings and reduce the risk for relapse. Whether you crave cigarettes, alcohol, sugary snacks, drugs, or gambling, exercise can help. One study of moderately heavy smokers who had abstained from smoking for 15 hours showed that even when faced with smoking-related images that would typically trigger cravings, the smokers had less desire to light up after exercising.[16]

8. **Get adequate sleep.** Have you ever noticed that after a night with almost no sleep, you wake up ravenously hungry and want to eat anything and everything in sight? That is because lack of sleep increases food cravings and cravings for other addictive behaviors. When you sleep well, your brain cleans itself and reinforces memory and learning in preparation for the next day, leading to better decision-making.

9. **Take natural supplements for craving control.** N-acetyl-cysteine, alpha-lipoic acid, and chromium are three natural supplements that can help take the edge off cravings. Here's how they work.

☐ *N-acetyl-cysteine (NAC):* NAC is an amino acid that is needed to produce glutathione, a powerful antioxidant. NAC binds to and removes dangerous toxic elements within the cells. Recently, NAC has been studied as a treatment for drug addiction because it functions to restore levels of the excitatory neurotransmitter glutamate in the reward center of the brain.[17] A growing body of research has found that NAC can reduce cravings for cocaine, heroin, and cigarettes and decrease the risk for relapse. It also reduces compulsive behavior in pathological gamblers and may be helpful in reducing food cravings. In one study, researchers conducted a double-blind placebo-controlled clinical trial on NAC and its effects on 27 pathological gamblers. After the eight-week trial, 83 percent of those taking NAC compared to only 29 percent of placebo takers experienced at least a 30 percent reduction in addictive behavior.[18] The typical adult dose is 600–1,200 mg twice a day to curb cravings.

☐ *Alpha-lipoic acid:* Made naturally in the body, alpha-lipoic acid may protect against cell damage in a variety of conditions. Strong evidence indicates that alpha-lipoic acid supports stable blood-sugar levels. Studies have shown that it improves insulin sensitivity and may be effective in treating type 2 diabetes.[19] The typical recommended adult dose is 100 mg twice a day.

☐ *Chromium:* Chromium picolinate is a nutritional supplement used to aid the body in the regulation of insulin, which enhances metabolism of glucose and fat. A strong link exists between depression, decreased insulin sensitivity, and diabetes. Supplementation with chromium picolinate effectively modulates carbohydrate cravings and appetite, which is beneficial to managing both the diabetes and depression. The typical recommended adult dosage is 200–600 micrograms a day.

HALT is a common acronym in addiction recovery circles for relapse prevention. Do not let yourself get too *hungry* (low blood sugar is associated with low blood flow to the PFC and more bad decisions), *angry* (anger lowers PFC function), *lonely* (being disconnected from others increases bad decisions), or *tired* (lack of sleep is associated with low PFC function). All of these factors impair decision-making skills and your ability to control cravings.

***Step 7: Drip dopamine; stop dumping it to keep your pleasure centers healthy.*** **B**

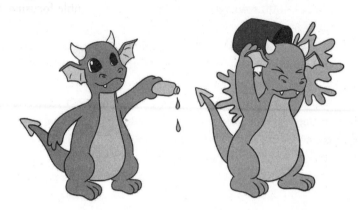

Dopamine is a feel-good chemical that our Addicted Dragons crave. Whenever we do something enjoyable, it's like pressing a button in the brain to release a little bit of dopamine to make us feel pleasure. If we push these pleasure buttons too often or too strongly, we reduce dopamine's effectiveness and wear out our pleasure centers. Eventually, it takes more and more excitement and stimulation to feel anything at all. Cocaine, methamphetamines, alcohol, and nicotine all cause dopamine surges that make these substances highly desirable—sometimes even more desirable than the things we need to survive like food, water, and sex. When people take drugs, the amount of dopamine released can be two to ten times more than what their brain produces for natural rewards.

Drugs and alcohol aren't the only substances that can hijack your brain. Playing video games, gambling, and looking at internet pornography can produce the same effect. So can certain foods. In *The End of Overeating*, former FDA commissioner Dr. David Kessler writes that the high-fat, high-sugar combinations found in many mouthwatering snacks light up the brain's dopamine pathway similar to the way drugs and alcohol do. He suggests that some people can actually get hooked on chocolate chip cookies the way other people get addicted to cocaine. Kessler and his team of researchers have seen this theory at work in animals too. In one study, they found that rats will work increasingly hard for a high-fat, high-sugar milkshake and that they will consume greater quantities of it if more sugar is added.[20]

Parkinson's disease teaches us a lot about dopamine because cells in an area of the brain called the substantia nigra, which produce dopamine, start to die, causing people to lose control over their muscle movements (shaking, stiffness, difficulty walking, balance). Low dopamine levels are also associated with depression, lack of motivation, low energy, and trouble focusing. One of my college professors, a very proper, loving man, developed a Parkinson's-like syndrome. When I treated him decades later, he loved Dr. Phil and Jerry Springer, which horrified his family. The conflict-driven television shows likely increased his dopamine levels, making him feel more alive.

The concept is simple. When we eat a bowl of fresh berries or hold our spouse's hand, our brains release small amounts of dopamine, which make us feel good. I call that dripping dopamine. It won't drain the dopamine stores in our brain. When we do a line of cocaine, watch porn, or eat caramel fudge brownies, our brains pump out lots of dopamine, which makes us feel great. That dumps dopamine, which can drain our dopamine stores, and increases the relative importance or salience of cocaine, porn, and caramel fudge brownies in our minds. Soon we no longer get much pleasure from eating berries or holding our spouse's hand and begin craving cocaine, porn, or caramel fudge brownies instead. Here is an illustration of the addiction cycle.

## THE ADDICTION CYCLE

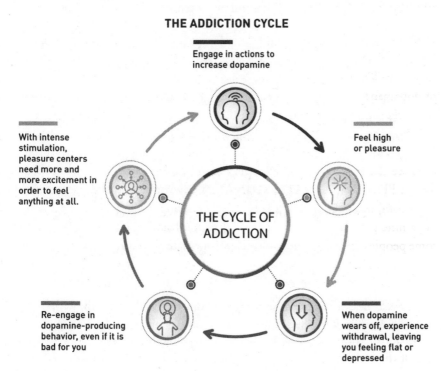

HOW TO PROTECT YOUR PLEASURE CENTERS

Some simple actions will help you protect your pleasure centers and keep them healthy. They involve dripping dopamine, a constant stream of small amounts, versus dumping dopamine, where you release a large amount all at once. Dumping dopamine wears out your pleasure centers.

- Limit low-value dopamine activities, such as caffeine, nicotine, excessive television, video games, undisciplined digital behavior, and scary movies.

- Limit activities that dump dopamine, including skydiving, motorcycle racing, heli-skiing, running with bulls, drug and alcohol use, porn, sugar.

- Engage in high-value dopamine activities that drip dopamine, such as sunlight (vitamin D), exercise, meditation, yoga, massage therapy, pleasurable music, hugs and hand-holding, and regular physical exercise, especially something you love that does not endanger your brain, such as dancing, swimming, or tennis.

- Make time to laugh—humor enhances the pleasure centers without wearing them out.

- Connect meaningful activities and pleasure, such as volunteering for activities you love. One example: I love table tennis and enjoy keeping score for others during tournaments.

- Start every day by thinking of three things for which you are grateful (a small dopamine drip) and one person you appreciate (another small dopamine drip), then reach out to tell that person you appreciate them with a text or email. You are building a bridge of gratitude, and if they respond, it is yet another, maybe bigger, dopamine drip.

- Seek pleasure in the little things in your life, such as a walk with a friend, holding hands with your spouse, a great meal, or a meaningful church service.

- Eat foods that contain dopamine-boosting properties, such as chicken, turkey, seafood, almonds, pumpkin and sesame seeds, turmeric, oregano, vegetables (for folate and magnesium), olive oil, and green tea (careful not to consume too much caffeinated tea).

- Consider supplements to support dopamine, such as omega-3 fatty acids, SAMe, L-tyrosine, magnesium, bacopa, and green tea extract.

| OTHER POSITIVE THINGS THAT DRIP DOPAMINE | OTHER NEGATIVE THINGS THAT DUMP DOPAMINE |
|---|---|
| Meaning and purpose | Jumping out of airplanes |
| Lasting love | Repeatedly falling in love |
| Digital discipline | High-risk sports (e.g., heli-skiing) |
| Relationships | Marital affairs |
| New learning | Excessive video games |
| Traveling | Pornography |
| Spiritual experience | Cocaine |
| Petting a puppy or kitten | Methamphetamines |
| Winning by striving to be your best | Winning by hurting others |
| Losing (when it motivates practice) | Gossiping |

*Step 8: Eliminate the Dragon Pushers and Users who make you vulnerable.* Ⓢ

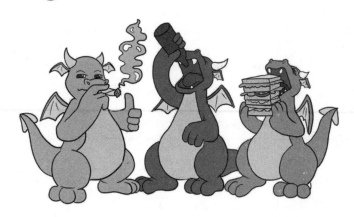

Cultivating bad habits—and good ones—is a team sport. You become like the people you spend time with. Dragon Pushers and Users are people who encourage or are complicit with your negative behaviors. Addictions need lots of accomplices to start and sustain them. Friends, mentors, or coaches are people who support your positive behaviors. Ask for their help. In my work with The Daniel Plan, a program I created with Pastor Rick Warren and Dr. Mark Hyman to help people get healthy through thousands of religious organizations, we found that adding friends improves your chances for success up to 40 percent, and this is especially true for drug addictions, weight loss, and fitness.

Identify your five most powerful friends who will support your good behaviors and five Dragon Pushers and Users who make it more likely you will not succeed in beating your addiction. Spend more time with the people who will help you. Consider talking to your Dragon Pushers and Users. If they are not interested or willing to help you, stop spending time around them if possible.

If you want to change your behavior, you need to stop seeing your Dragon Pushers and Users or somehow turn them into friends. Some Dragon Pushers and Users can become friends if you have crucial conversations with them. Explain what they can start doing to help you, what they can stop doing, and what they can continue doing. Some don't even realize that they are influencing you to make poor choices and will want to help once they understand your goals to kick addiction.

## ARE THESE PEOPLE FRIENDS OR DRAGON PUSHERS AND USERS?

- Spouse
- Children
- Parents
- Grandparents
- Siblings
- In-laws
- Aunts, uncles, cousins
- Friends
- Neighbors
- Bosses
- Coworkers
- Teachers
- Classmates
- Students
- School administrators
- Church members or staff
- Support group participants
- Community club members

Riz had no problem sticking with his new eating regimen until he went to dinner parties with friends and family. Then his loved ones would offer him all kinds of foods and alcoholic drinks that he used to love but that didn't fit into his new brain-healthy lifestyle. Riz's friends and family would try to pressure and coax him into eating or drinking things he had given up. "What's wrong with you?" they would ask. "You're not obese. Why aren't you having any kebab? Why aren't you eating any rice? You've always loved kebab and rice." They made Riz feel like he was being rude if he didn't give in and take a helping . . . or two.

I know that feeling very well. When I became a grandfather for the first time, I couldn't wait to visit my new grandson, Elias. When I went to my daughter's home, a friend of mine was also visiting. She asked me if I wanted something to eat, and I said no, I wasn't hungry. A few minutes later, she asked me again, and I told her no again. I thought that would be the end of that discussion, but she continued to ask me an additional five times if I wanted something to eat!

You will face many types of Dragon Pushers who will attempt to derail your health efforts. Do not let other people make you fat, stupid, and unhappy!

### Don't let Dragon Pushers sabotage your health

Dragon Pushers are the people or organizations that threaten to derail your efforts to get and stay healthy. Here are some tips on how to deal with Dragon Pushers:

1. If you are going to a dinner with friends or family, call ahead to inform the host that you are on a special brain-healthy diet and won't be drinking alcohol or eating certain foods. You only have to do this once or twice before your friends start to ask you what they could serve that is brain-healthy.

2. When going to parties, consider eating something ahead of time so you won't be hungry or tempted by alcohol at the event.

3. Be up front with Dragon Pushers. Explain that you are trying to eat a more balanced diet or stay away from alcohol and drugs, and that when they offer you cake, chips, pizza, or alcohol or marijuana, it makes it more difficult for you.

4. Instead of going out to lunch or happy hour with friends, choose activities that aren't centered around food or alcohol, such as going for a walk.

5. When people offer seconds (food or drink), tell them you are finished. If they insist, explain that you are watching your health. If they continue to push you, gently ask them why they don't want you to be healthy.

6. Avoid visiting with coworkers who have a bowl of candy on their desk.

7. Eat very slowly so when the host starts asking guests if they want seconds, you can say you are still working on your first helping. By the time you have finished, the second round of eating could be over, and you won't have to be subjected to the offer for more.

8. Commit to taking control of your own body and don't let other people steal your mind.

9. Tell restaurant servers "no bread" or "no alcohol" when seated.

10. Inform parents and in-laws ahead of time that you won't be partaking in certain foods or drinks at family gatherings.

11. Bring a sack lunch instead of eating out or eating at the cafeteria.

12. If alcohol is a problem, don't meet friends at a bar.

13. Avoid associating with acquaintances who engage in the addictive behaviors you are trying to quit.

14. Unsubscribe from any online gambling or sports-betting sites if that's a problem for you.

15. Remove yourself from any group chats or texts with fellow gamers if you are trying to limit your game playing.

*Step 9: Tame your Dragons from the Past and kill the ANTs.* Ⓟ

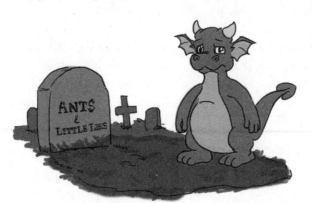

To get and stay free of Addicted Dragons, you have to tame your Dragons from the Past and kill the ANTs you tell yourself. Corinne, 52, had smoked since she was a teenager. By the time she came to see me, she had been smoking for almost 40 years, and she had the wrinkled skin and breathing problems to prove it. Her loved ones desperately wanted her to stop smoking. Corinne wanted to quit but didn't believe she could do it. "I can't stop," she told me in one of our first sessions.

Corinne had started smoking after her mother, who also smoked, abandoned her to run off with a new boyfriend, leaving Corinne with an aunt to raise her. As a teen, Corinne felt so much anxiety that her aunt would also abandon her that she used smoking to soothe herself. The Anxious Dragons continued to haunt her throughout her life. To quit smoking, Corinne would have to tame her Anxious Dragons and kill the ANTs that kept her addicted to cigarettes. We worked together on her anxiety, and we tackled her "I can't stop smoking" ANT using the five questions you learned about in section 3.

ANT: *I can't stop smoking.*

1. Is it true? Yes.

2. Can you absolutely know it's true? Initially, she said yes; she knew she couldn't do it. Then she thought about it and said, "Of course, I can't know for sure, especially if I got the right help."

3. How do you feel when you have the thought? "I feel powerless, sad, weak-willed, stupid, out of control, like a bad influence on my children."

4. Who would you be without the thought? "I would be hopeful, optimistic, more likely to give it my best effort."

5. Turnaround: What is the opposite thought? Is it truer than the original thought? "I can stop smoking." She thought about this for a while and said that if she got help and really tried, it could be true. Then she felt a sense of control and committed to a program.

Corinne eventually did stop smoking and felt better than ever. Controlling her ANTs and Dragons from the Past were critical steps in the process.

***Step 10: Get help from those who have tamed their own Addicted Dragons.*** **S**

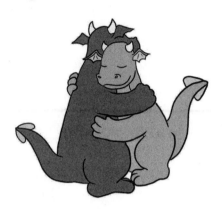

Success leaves clues. Addiction mentors and support groups are often critical pieces to the healing process. The people you meet at support groups have walked your path and may have strategies that can help you. Other people who have struggled with your issue can help you feel less lonely and give you an outlet to express your thoughts. Often just hearing what you are thinking out loud, with the input of others, can help eliminate many of your ANTs. Research shows that support groups can decrease anxiety and depression. They can help you stay motivated to stick to a new way of living. They can give you hope. They are also an affordable and often free way of getting help.

Choose your helpers wisely. As we've seen, you become like the dragons you spend time with. Choose people who represent how you want to live, not those who increase your risk of relapse. Here are some tips to choosing mentors or support groups:

1. Pick people who've been successful at taming dragons like yours. The longer they've kept the dragons at bay, the better.

2. Pick people who will tell you the truth with kindness. Sugarcoating is not helpful (and you know what I think of sugar), but neither is being condescending or mean.

3. Don't be afraid of those who are younger than you.

4. Choose people who will challenge you.

5. Choose people with similar values.

6. Choose people with two ears and one mouth, who take time to listen.

7. Choose people you are not afraid to call or text.

8. Once you choose someone, be open to their input but also evaluate it. Don't be so open-minded your brain falls out of your skull. That is how cults start.

9. Meet mentors at in-person or online support groups, through mutual friends, church, or other organizations. Be kind to everyone you meet because you never know when a mentor will appear.

10. Take an interest in those you respect. Most people who ask for mentoring are only interested in themselves. The best way to put off a mentor is to do it in a self-centered way. Finding a great mentor begins when you take an interest in someone you respect. Then consider how you can add value to their lives. That way you don't have to ask them to mentor you, but they volunteer.

---

*The fastest way to get healthy is to find the healthiest person you can stand and spend as much time around him or her as possible.*

---

## CREATE YOUR OWN BRAIN-HEALTH SUPPORT NETWORK

Relationships help you thrive and can keep you on track toward your goals. Research has demonstrated that strong relationships are associated with health, happiness, and success. The health of your peer group is one of the strongest predictors of your health and longevity. This exercise will help you create and sustain your own network.

# CREATE YOUR OWN
# BRAIN HEALTH SUPPORT NETWORK

Relationships help you thrive and can help keep you on track toward your goals. Research has demonstrated that strong relationships are associated with health, happiness and success. The health of your peer group is one of the strongest predictors of your health and longevity. This exercise will help you create and sustain your own network.

*Write down 10 relationships that are*
*potentially supportive to you and your health.*

1. _____
2. _____
3. _____
4. _____
5. _____
6. _____
7. _____
8. _____
9. _____
10. _____

*Of those above, write down the top five and how*
*they may be supportive of your health.*

NAME                IN WHAT AREA CAN THEY BE HELPFUL?

1. _____    _____
2. _____    _____
3. _____    _____
4. _____    _____
5. _____    _____

# AN IN-DEPTH LOOK AT
# MY BRAIN-HEALTH SUPPORT NETWORK

*Who (initials)? What wisdom do they have?*

1. _____
2. _____
3. _____
4. _____
5. _____

*Who (initials)? How can I help them?*

1. _____
2. _____
3. _____
4. _____
5. _____

*Who (initials)? How can they help me?*

1. _____
2. _____
3. _____
4. _____
5. _____

# WHO ELSE COULD BE PLUGGED INTO
# MY BRAIN-HEALTH SUPPORT NETWORK?

*Who? What wisdom do they have? How I can help them?*
*How can they help me?*

1. _____
2. _____
3. _____
4. _____
5. _____

***Step 11: List the people your Addicted Dragons have hurt, share it with a mentor or sponsor, and make amends if you can.*** **S** **SP**

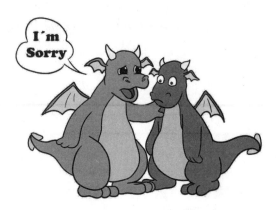

This is a combination of AA steps that is essential to improve your relationships and to have a better sense of yourself—let's do this step with a better-balanced brain. None of us exists in a vacuum. Admitting your wrongs to others, asking for forgiveness, and making amends if you're able can help free you from the Should and Shaming Dragons and make it less likely to continue the behavior that is hurtful to others.

### JOSE AND ANGELA

I once got a call from a producer at the *Dr. Phil Show* who asked if I would help with a program on infidelity. They wanted me to evaluate and perform SPECT scans on Jose, a compulsive cheater.[21] Jose and his wife, Angela, were struggling with his infidelity, lies, and pornography addiction. In just four years, Jose had cheated on Angela eight times. On the show, Dr. Phil put those eight instances into perspective: "My dad used to say, 'For every rat you see, there are 50 you don't.'"

Within three months of getting married, Angela found out Jose was cheating on her. In fact, he had been with another girl when he asked her to marry him, during their wedding planning, and right after Angela had a baby girl.

"I was devastated and very angry," Angela said. "I gave my gun to my mom because I thought I was going to shoot him. After I took Jose back, I found out that he has cheated on me with numerous girls."

Jose said, "I have always been the kind of guy to just hook up when someone comes along. I was out of the home for about five weeks until we decided to patch things up."

Jose admitted that before he got married, he never felt guilt. After all, his father cheated on his mom. "I'm worried that I have a sexual addiction because I have a need for something stimulating," he said, whether that be affairs, fast cars, or living on the edge. Jose was an adrenaline junkie, who had a high need for speed, along with excitement-seeking behavior. He lost his driver's license after getting four speeding tickets. Though he said he'd been faithful to Angela in the past year, he had a problem with pornography.

On the show, Dr. Phil asked Jose, "If this is your proclivity, why not get a divorce and go do what you wanted to do?" Jose replied that he wanted a wife and a family. His father's behavior had a negative effect on his family. Jose wanted something different: to be a positive influence for his daughter. Jose wanted help, and he wanted to stop hurting the people he loved. Going on the show was his way of making amends and proving to his wife that he was serious about changing his behavior.

His brain SPECT scan showed three highly significant abnormalities.

1. Increased activity in the anterior cingulate gyrus, which is the brain's gear shifter, often associated with compulsive behavior. In addition to cheating, Jose compulsively got tattoos and was covered head to toe, which had prevented him from getting many jobs he wanted.

2. Decreased activity in the PFC, his Dragon Tamer.

3. A head injury pattern. Jose's scan clearly showed evidence of brain trauma, with areas damaged in the front and back parts of his brain.

**HEALTHY SURFACE SPECT SCAN**

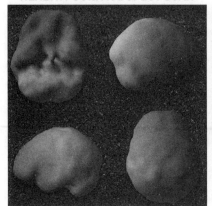

Full, even, symmetrical activity

**JOSE'S SURFACE SPECT SCAN**

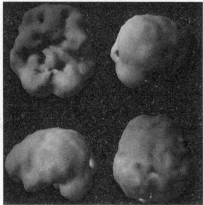

Decreased activity in the front (prefrontal cortex) and the back of the brain consistent with a prior brain injury(s)

**HEALTHY ACTIVE SPECT SCAN**

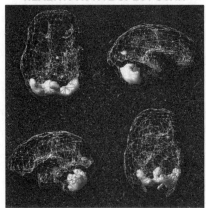

Highest activity at back of brain

**JOSE'S ACTIVE SPECT SCAN**

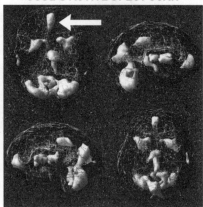

Increased anterior cingulate activity in front part of the brain consistent with trouble shifting attention (arrow)

Initially, I asked Jose if he had ever had a brain injury. He said no. But I knew better. I've scanned tens of thousands of patients with brain injuries, so I persisted. Again he said no. I have heard this same story from so many patients that we joke about it at the Amen Clinics. We see the obvious pattern of a brain injury on their scans but they never think of how they may have hit their heads.

"Ever play a contact sport?" I asked.

"Yes," he said. "I played football in high school." He then told me about how many times he had concussions. Next, he mentioned that he was a bull rider and a mixed martial artist. He had been hit hard in the head many times. Then, quietly he said, "And I am a head banger."

"Excuse me?" I responded.

Embarrassed but smiling, Jose said, "I used to break things with my head. It was like a party trick. I could break cans and beer bottles with my forehead." Then he added, "When I got drunk, I often put dents in doors and walls with my head. I can usually find the studs in the walls with my head."

Angela was angry. She wanted Jose to do something to change. She thought he could use willpower. Angela said, "Unless I see a complete change, I am done."

On the show, Jose said he was excited to see the results of the scans. In his no-nonsense Texas drawl, Dr. Phil said, "It is odd to hear someone say they are excited to have brain damage. You think this gives you a pass. It is like, 'Hey, it's not my fault, my brain's not right.'"

Jose then said something very profound, "I am not thinking of this as an excuse, but I am hoping this might be a key to help change my behavior."

The show took an interesting twist. Dr. Phil asked the audience what they thought about sexual addiction: Was it a real biological phenomenon or an excuse for bad behavior? The audience's opinion was that it was an excuse. Yet from the brain scans I have seen and my years of experience in helping people unravel from addictions, I know strong brain issues are at play. I have seen sexual addictions ruin people's lives and bring many addicts to the point of financial ruin and even suicide. I also believe that addictions, including sexual addictions, are going to get worse in our society as we are wearing out the brain's pleasure centers with the constant exposure to highly stimulating activities, such as video games, text messaging, sexting, internet pornography, scary movies, and highly addictive foods like cinnamon rolls and double cheeseburgers.

After the show, Jose and Angela agreed to see me for help. It was another way Jose showed her that he wanted to make amends. He was in enough pain that he was willing to follow my recommendations. Here was his prescription:

**Stop drinking alcohol.** Alcohol lowers Jose's prefrontal cortex capacity and decreases his brain's braking power to help him say no to his urges.

**Get enough sleep to maintain healthy brain function.** Getting less than six hours of sleep at night has been associated with lower overall blood flow to the brain, which means more bad decisions.

**Clean up his diet.** Only eat healthy food that serves his optimal brain function. Eat multiple times a day to keep his blood sugar stable.

**Eliminate the caffeine and energy drinks that were a staple of his diet.** Caffeine constricts blood flow to the brain. Anything that lowers or constricts blood flow to the brain increases bad decision-making.

**Supplement his brain.** Jose was an impulsive-compulsive addict. I added rhodiola and green tea to help with his impulsivity and 5-HTP and saffron to help with his compulsions. I also added nutrients to help his overall brain health, including a multiple vitamin/mineral supplement and omega-3 fatty acids.

Over the next seven months, I regularly saw Jose and Angela to monitor their progress. In our sessions, we discussed his nutrition, supplements, and strategies to control his urges, which were becoming less and less powerful. I had Jose plant two words in his head—*Then what?*—to help boost his prefrontal cortex by thinking about the future consequences of his behavior. It finally clicked when he heard the chorus of the Clay Walker song "Then What?" Jose realized that if he didn't ask, "Then what?" and make new, better choices, he was going to be somebody who "ain't anybody any body's gonna trust."[22]

Things were going so well for Jose and Angela that they started to discuss having another child. They went to Hawaii on vacation to talk more about their future together. While there, Jose saw people jumping off a 60-foot cliff into the water below. His immediate reaction was that he wanted to do it too. Being a thrill seeker had been part of his life for a very long time. Some would say it was part of his DNA. As Jose hiked up the hillside, Angela rolled her eyes, thinking yet again to herself, *He is such a show-off.* She had seen him do so many stupid things throughout their time together. Would it ever end?

When Jose got to the top of the cliff and looked down, something happened in his mind. He started to feel uncomfortable, even anxious. Although he saw other people jumping off the cliff, he could not clearly see the rocks jutting up in the water in order to avoid them. He thought to himself, *Then what? What if I land wrong? What if I get hurt? What if I am paralyzed? I have a wife and child, and we want another child. Being paralyzed will not help any of us. Do I really need to do this?*

He stepped out of line to think about his next move. This level of thought, pausing to contemplate the consequences of a risky action, was new for Jose. After a minute or so, he decided not to jump. With a sense of freedom, he began walking down the hillside. Angela was stunned. She had never seen Jose do anything like that before. Maybe there was hope.

Shortly after the trip to Hawaii, when they told me this story, I had to see his brain. We did a follow-up SPECT scan on Jose, which showed dramatic improvement from seven months earlier. With enhanced brain health, he had started thinking more about how his actions would affect Angela, an important aspect of making amends.

**JOSE'S FIRST SPECT SCAN**

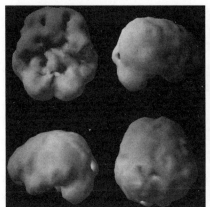

Decreased activity in the front (prefrontal cortex) and the back of the brain consistent with a prior brain injury(s)

**JOSE'S FOLLOW-UP SPECT SCAN
7 MONTHS LATER**

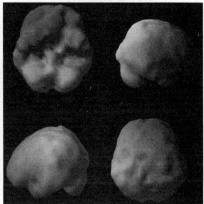

Overall dramatic improvement

By working the treatment plan, Jose literally changed his brain and dramatically improved and likely extended his life and his marriage. Jose could have apologized and tried to make amends for the rest of his life. But if we didn't first fix his brain, it would have never lasted. Jose has been sober for 10 years and recently finished his nurse anesthetist program. I am so proud of him.

*Step 12: Carry the message of brain health to others and continue to practice these 12 steps.* (S) (SP)

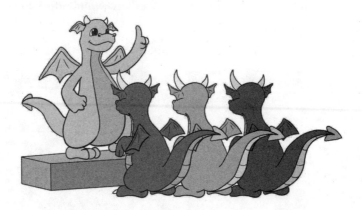

This last step is similar to the 12th Step of AA and other anonymous programs. If you want to keep your sobriety, you need to share the principles with others. It completely works for brain health, too. Your brain is always listening to what you do, but it is also listening to the actions of others. Make sure you are sharing brain health, not illness, with those you love.

Get it, give it away, and keep it forever. This a mantra I learned after creating The Daniel Plan with my friends Pastor Rick Warren and Dr. Mark Hyman. If you want to keep your health, you have to learn how to do it and then give it away to others. It is in the act of giving that you create your own support group, making it more likely you will stay on the program.

Whenever Tana and I are on the Saddleback Church campus, we hear story after story of how The Daniel Plan has changed lives:

- "My numbers are so much better!
  - Cholesterol was 202, now it is 164.
  - Blood pressure was 142/92, now it is 125/75.
  - Body mass index was 35.7, now it is 26.1."

- "No more headaches! It's amazing. I was taking prescription pain medication almost daily. It's been more than two weeks without any pain or pills!"

- "My mood is so much more stable and positive."

- "With the elimination of sugar, flour, salt, and processed foods, I rarely have any cravings and have found I eat smaller amounts of nutrient-rich foods."

- "Ninety-eight percent of my headaches at night have disappeared. I wake up feeling clearheaded instead of foggy."

- "I don't have body, joint, or muscle pain in the mornings."

- "I'm off my high blood-pressure meds . . . and am working on getting off of my type 2 diabetes and cholesterol meds."

- "Odd to say this in church, but my sex life has dramatically improved!"

Many people ask me what they can do if their children, families, or coworkers are not receptive to a new way of eating or behaving. My answer is always this: "You have to live the message." You cannot give something you do not live. Don't let others ever be your excuse to hurt yourself, listen to your Addicted Dragons, and not do the program.

If these 12 steps don't give you freedom from the Addicted Dragons, get a professional assessment and consider having someone look at your brain.

## 12 New Steps to Heal Addictions and the Circles They Address

**B P S SP** • Step 1: Know what you want.

**P S** • Step 2: Know when your Addicted Dragons have taken you hostage.

**B** • Step 3: Make a decision to care for, balance, and repair your brain.

**B P S SP** • Step 4: Reach for forgiveness for yourself and others.

**B** • Step 5: Know your Addicted Dragon's brain type.

(B) (P) • Step 6: Lock up the Craving Dragons.

(B) • Step 7: Drip dopamine; stop dumping it to keep your pleasure centers healthy.

(S) • Step 8: Eliminate the Dragon Pushers and Users who make you vulnerable.

(P) • Step 9: Tame your Dragons from the Past and kill the ANTs.

(S) • Step 10: Get help from those who have tamed their own Addicted Dragons.

(S) (SP) • Step 11: List the people your Addicted Dragons have hurt, share it with a mentor or sponsor, and make amends if you can.

(S) (SP) • Step 12: Carry the message of brain health to others and continue to practice these 12 steps.

SECTION 7

# THE DRAGON TAMER

IS YOURS HEALTHY, WEAK, OR OVERCONTROLLING?

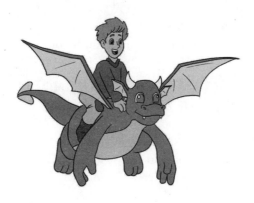

The brain is a sneaky organ. We all have weird, crazy, stupid, sexual, violent thoughts that no one should ever hear. During the first few months of the pandemic when toilet paper and paper towels became the hottest commodities, did you ever go to the grocery store and see someone with armloads of TP and paper towels and wonder what it would be like to trip them just to see the stuff fly everywhere? Am I the only person? Of course, I'd never actually trip someone. My Dragon Tamer, housed in the front third of my brain in the prefrontal cortex (PFC), protects me from impulses that seem to pop up from nowhere. To keep the dragons and ANTs we've met and will meet from stealing your happiness, leading you toward bad habits, and destroying your relationships, you must strengthen and protect your Dragon Tamer.

## YOUR DRAGON TAMER: IS IT STRONG, WEAK, OR OVERCONTROLLING?

The PFC, your Dragon Tamer, is the leader of the four circles of health: biological, psychological, social, and spiritual, which I introduced on page 12. If your Dragon Tamer is weak, your dragons will run wild and destroy one or more of the circles. If your Dragon Tamer is overcontrolling, you are more likely to obsess about your dragons and micromanage them, leading them to get worse. When your Dragon Tamer is strong and healthy, your dragons will play nicely with each other and help you achieve your goals. For example, when my dad died and I was filled with sadness in addition to the extra stress I was feeling from the pandemic, my dragons could have seized on this moment of weakness to start breathing fire on my brain. But by practicing the strategies in this book to keep my frontal lobes healthy—getting adequate sleep, eating brain-healthy foods, avoiding alcohol, and more—I was able to keep those dragons in their place. Having a healthy Dragon Tamer has helped me grieve in a healthy way rather than in a self-destructive way.

In this section, we will explore the functions of the Dragon Tamer, how to keep it strong, and what to do when it is weak or overcontrolling. We will also consider the ADHD Dragon, which can get out of control when the Dragon Tamer goes on vacation.

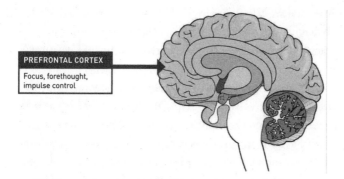

PREFRONTAL CORTEX
Focus, forethought, impulse control

## DRAGON TAMER DUTIES

The Dragon Tamer (PFC) acts as the brain's brake that prevents us from saying or doing stupid things. British comedian Dudley Moore once said, "The best car safety device is a rearview mirror with a cop in it." Your Dragon Tamer acts like the cop in your head, and like police officers who need constant training to stay sharp, it needs regular training to function at a high level and not have lapses that ruin your relationships.

The PFC is the most human, thoughtful part of the brain. It is larger in humans than any other animal: 30 percent of the human brain; 11 percent of the chimpanzee brain, our closest primate cousin; 7 percent of your dog's brain; 3 percent of the cat's brain, which is why felines need nine lives; and one percent of the mouse's brain, which is why cats eat mice.[1]

Here are the main functions of the PFC, or what I call Dragon Tamer duties:

- Supervision
- Protection from saying or doing stupid things
- Goal setting
- Goal-directed behavior
- Breaking through obstacles
- Persistence
- Planning
- Focus
- Forethought
- Judgment
- Impulse control
- Organization
- Empathy
- Insight

- Learning from mistakes
- Saying no to behaviors inconsistent with goals
- Conscientiousness—e.g., consistently showing up when you say you will

The PFC is the last part of the brain to develop. It is generally not finished maturing until people are in their mid to late twenties, which is why car insurance rates generally go down after the age of 25 as young adults start making better decisions. Knowing this, it is easier to understand why kids, teens, and young adults have lower executive function—81 percent of teens report failing to achieve an important goal they set for themselves. For older adults, understanding development can lead to more empathy, support, and supervision for young people. That's also why it is a parent's job to be their child's Dragon Tamer until theirs is fully developed. When your Dragon Tamer is healthy, it helps you match your behavior over time to reach your goals, even in periods of stress and uncertainty like the pandemic. When it is weak, it is more vulnerable in high-stress situations, and when children are left unsupervised, you never know what awful things may happen.

---

*As a parent, your job is to be your child's Dragon Tamer until theirs is fully developed.*

---

The PFC is called the "executive brain" because it acts like the boss at work to supervise the employees and tasks that need to be done for the business to be successful. The PFC also sends signals to other parts of the brain to calm them down, such as the Dragons from the Past and the ANTs that attack you. When the Dragon Tamer is healthy, it is like a conductor in an orchestra that gets the musicians to play together to create beautiful music.

The Dragon Tamer also acts as the brain's conscience, helping you match your behavior over time to reach your goals in a manner consistent with your morals and beliefs. I think of the PFC like Jiminy Cricket from the movie *Pinocchio*. Who was Jiminy Cricket? Pinocchio's conscience. What was his role? He helped Pinocchio reach his goal to be a real boy. When Jiminy Cricket was lost to Pinocchio, the wooden puppet almost died from the bad decisions he made.

Unless you are asleep, your Dragon Tamer (PFC) is always watching you, protecting you from your impulses and the first thoughts that come into your head. Sleep causes the Dragon Tamer to go offline, which is why your dreams are often unconstrained and wild.

# WEAK DRAGON TAMER PROBLEMS WHEN THE PFC IS TOO LOW IN ACTIVITY

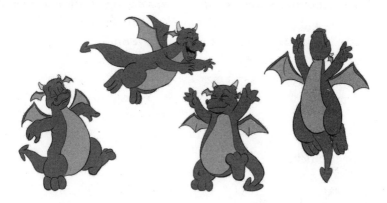

When the Dragon Tamer is off duty, on vacation, hurt, or sick, life becomes much harder for you and everyone in your life. When the PFC is low in activity, your emotional brain and the Dragons from the Past are more likely to torture you (emotional circle); your ANTs are more likely to attack you (psychological circle); and your decision-making can cause big trouble for you (in any of the four circles). In the days when the coronavirus was prompting most people to shelter at home, the people with weak Dragon Tamers were flocking to the beaches and cavorting at parties. Low activity in the PFC is associated with:

- Lack of internal supervision
- Stupid words or actions
- Lack of goals
- Erratic behavior
- Inability to move past obstacles
- Lack of persistence
- Lack of planning
- Distractibility
- Little forethought
- Poor judgment
- Low impulse control
- Disorganization
- Low empathy
- Lack of insight
- Trouble learning from mistakes

Indeed, when the Dragon Tamer is off duty, you may have more fun initially. Research suggests that low activity in the PFC has been associated with feeling spontaneous and more creative (if you can just balance that without losing control and making good decisions overall). When the PFC activity is low and the Dragon Tamer is off duty, people have a much higher incidence of:

- School failure
- Divorce
- Job failure
- Legal issues
- Speeding tickets
- Incarceration
- Financial problems
- Excitement, conflict, or negative attention seeking
- Chronic lateness, poor time management
- Relapse from addiction programs
- Procrastination
- Saying yes too often
- Interrupting others
- Lack of conscientiousness
- Mental health issues, especially ADHD and addictions

You can see why protecting your Dragon Tamer is essential for a happier, healthier life.

## WHAT HURTS YOUR DRAGON TAMER

What hurts the PFC and dulls its ability to tame your dragons and eliminate ANTs? Many things in the biological circle of health, which is why I've written so much about the importance of brain health.[2] You must protect the part of the brain that protects you and pay attention to the following problems:

1. **Anything that lowers blood flow to the brain:** Blood is essential to life. It brings nourishment to every cell in your body and takes away waste. New research suggests that brain cells don't age; rather, it's your blood vessels that age![3] Anything that damages blood vessels damages your brain and starves it of the nutrients it needs. Low blood flow is the number one predictor of Alzheimer's disease and

is associated with ADHD, depression, and schizophrenia, a serious psychotic disorder. High blood pressure, any form of vascular or heart disease, lack of exercise, caffeine, and nicotine—lower blood flow and the function of the Dragon Tamer.

2. **Aging:** The older you get, the lower blood flow is to the PFC. Brain imaging clearly shows that your brain typically becomes less active with age. This is why the older you get, the more serious you need to be about taking care of your brain.

3. **Inflammation,** which comes from the Latin word meaning to set a fire, is like having a low-level fire destroying your organs. Having low levels of the omega-3 fatty acids EPA and DHA in your bloodstream is associated with inflammation and linked to ADHD, a sign of Dragon Tamer dysfunction.

4. **Head trauma:** This is the most common cause of Dragon Tamer problems. In one study my team published, 94 percent of head injuries affected the frontal lobes.[4] The brain is soft, about the consistency of soft butter, and your skull is really hard with multiple sharp boney ridges. So protect your brain from injury by avoiding any activities that could cause you to hit your head. (Note: Do not let your children play tackle football or hit soccer balls with their heads.)

5. **Toxins,** including mold, heavy metals like lead, or other environmental toxins can damage the Dragon Tamer. Drugs and alcohol lower blood flow and function to the Dragon Tamer, which is why people tend to make poorer decisions when they are high, stoned, or drunk.

6. **Obesity** has been shown to lower Dragon Tamer function because it causes inflammation in your body; protect your weight. (Read about the Overeating Bad Habit Dragon in section 4.)

7. **High and low blood sugar** can hurt the Dragon Tamer. High blood sugar (prediabetes and diabetes) damages blood vessels and lowers function of the PFC. Low blood sugar, from fasting or hypoglycemia, also lowers blood flow to the brain. The quality of your diet is critical to the health of your Dragon Tamer.

8. **Poor sleep,** including insomnia, sleep apnea, and sleeping pills, can take the Dragon Tamer off-line. An estimated 50 to 70 million Americans have sleep-related issues, according to the American Sleep Association.[5] When you sleep, your brain cleans or washes itself. If sleep is disrupted, trash builds up in your brain, which damages your memory. Getting less than seven hours of sleep at night decreases the strength of your Dragon Tamer and is associated with weight issues, hypertension, and accidents. It may also cause trouble in your marriage because you are more likely to say something you wish you hadn't.

## *Your Brain Is Always Listening to Your Blood Sugar Level*

### *TOO HIGH (HYPERGLYCEMIA)*

| | |
|---|---|
| Confusion | Seizures |
| Tiredness | Headaches |
| Thirst | Trouble concentrating |
| Hunger | Blurred vision |
| Shortness of breath | Weight loss |
| Stomach pain | |

### *TOO LOW (HYPOGLYCEMIA)*

| | |
|---|---|
| Sleepiness, feeling drugged | Anxiety/panic attacks |
| Mental confusion | Palpitations |
| Inability to concentrate | Shaky hands |
| Impaired memory | "Butterflies" in stomach |
| Dizziness, light-headedness | Flushing/sweating |
| | Faintness/fainting |
| Nervousness | Head pressure |
| Depression | Frontal headache |
| Irritability | Insomnia |
| Blurred vision | Abdominal pain/diarrhea |
| Overwhelming fatigue | |

## OVERCONTROLLING DRAGON TAMER PROBLEMS

While low activity in the PFC causes the Dragon Tamer to take a break and go on vacation, hyperactivity in the PFC (the scientific term is *hyperfrontality*) is associated with the Dragon Tamer always being on guard, worrying, obsessively thinking, micromanaging, and being upset when things don't go his or her way. Hyperfrontality has been associated with obsessive-compulsive disorder, obsessive-compulsive personality trait (being rigid and inflexible, and having excessive self-control), and some forms of depression[6]—all psychological and social issues that make your relationships more difficult. When the World Health Organization first announced that the coronavirus was indeed a global pandemic, people with an overcontrolling Dragon Tamer were the ones hoarding toilet paper, paper towels, hand sanitizer, water, and canned food.

My patient Mark, 42, had an overactive PFC. He was a high-performing CEO at a technology start-up. His investors were excited about the potential of his business, but it had a very high employee turnover. A consultant reported to the board of directors that he believed Mark was micromanaging the team, causing them to feel demoralized. One of the board members recommended Mark come to see me.

After first resisting, Mark told me he had family members who suffered from alcohol abuse, depression, and obsessive-compulsive disorder. His grandfather was famous for holding grudges for decades. Mark's Active SPECT scan showed significant increased activity in his PFC. This pattern made him more vulnerable to being rigid, worrying, holding grudges, and micromanaging his employees. When he understood his brain was causing his social problems and agitating some of his dragons, he agreed to take some simple supplements, saffron and 5HTP, and increase his exercise to help calm this part of the brain. Over the next year, the turnover in his company decreased and the board was much happier with his performance.

**HEALTHY VS. HYPERFRONTAL ACTIVE SPECT SCANS**

Healthy                                    Hyperfrontal

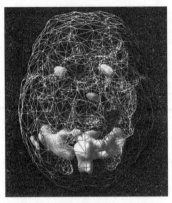
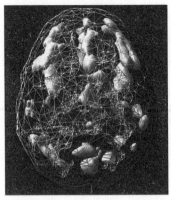

White equals most active parts of the brain,        Excessive activity in the front
typically in cerebellum in back, bottom area              where the PFC sits

## ARE THE ADHD DRAGONS RUINING YOUR LIFE?

When the Dragon Tamer is tired, weak, or on vacation, people often exhibit signs of ADHD, also called attention deficit disorder (ADD). Undiagnosed ADHD ruins people's lives. It is associated with low activity in the PFC. Its hallmark symptoms[7] are:

- Short attention for regular, routine, everyday things: They struggle to focus on activities such as homework, paperwork, and chores.
- Distractibility: They tend to see too much, hear too much, and sense too much, which distracts them from whatever task they need to get done.
- Disorganization of time and space: They are often late, and their homes, rooms, desks, and book bags can be a mess.
- Procrastination: They tend to get things done at the very last minute.
- Impulse control issues: They tend to do or say things without fully thinking them through.

If you can relate to these symptoms, consider getting diagnosed and treated. ADHD is associated with all of the Dragon Tamer problems listed above. Treatment can dramatically improve the quality of your life, work, and relationships.

## *Jessica*

Jessica, 38, had felt depressed since the birth of her third child. She was a nurse who was married to a professional soccer player. He had been traded a number of times, and they had moved 13 times over eight years. She was chronically overwhelmed, causing stress in her marriage and with the kids. She had been in therapy for years, but it never seemed to help enough. Her primary care doctor put her on Lexapro (a selective serotonin reuptake inhibitor) to boost the neurotransmitter serotonin in her brain. Serotonin tends to calm brain activity, which is helpful if the brain works too hard but very bad for the brain if it is underactive. Lexapro had made Jessica much worse, disinhibiting her and causing her to say mean, hurtful things to her husband and children.

Jessica's SPECT scan showed lower overall activity in her brain, especially in the PFC, which is a classic finding in people with ADHD. Giving her Lexapro was one of the worst interventions her doctor could have prescribed. As I gathered more history, I learned that Jessica had been a good student but that teachers said she had talked too much, was restless, and had trouble sitting still. Homework had taken her twice as long as it took her friends. She was often late and disorganized. As a nurse, she used a lot of caffeine to stay awake and focused. She likely inherited her ADHD from her mother, who was impulsive, irritable, chronically disorganized, and usually late. Jessica had classic untreated ADHD, causing stress not only for herself but also for her husband and children. Her Dragon Tamer had been weak her whole life. And the multiple moves put Jessica under chronic stress so she could never relax.

When I treated her ADHD with nutrients, including omega-3 fatty acids and zinc, and a low dose of a stimulant, her focus improved, her stress lessened, and her marriage was dramatically better. Her brain also became much healthier. Initially, Jessica did not want to take medicine because she did not want to be someone different. I told her the medicine and supplements wouldn't make her a different person, but they would help her be who she really was when her brain worked right. Strengthening her Dragon Tamer helped everyone in her family.

**JESSICA'S SURFACE SPECT SCAN BEFORE AND AFTER TREATMENT**

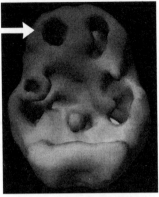
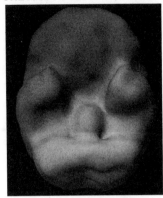

Before: underside surface                         After: underside surface
Very low PFC activity                               Marked improvement

## STRENGTHEN YOUR DRAGON TAMER TO MAKE GOOD DECISIONS

The first and most important step to strengthening your Dragon Tamer is to know what you want, to clearly and concisely define the goals for your life. Then ask yourself every day, *Does my behavior get me what I want?* Without doing this, your behavior will often be driven by the Scheming Dragons we mentioned in section 5. Tell your PFC what you want, and it will help you match your behavior to get it! Your brain makes happen what it sees. If you focus on negativity, you will feel depressed. If you focus on fear, you are likely to feel anxious. If you focus on achieving your goals, you are much more likely to reach them. Too many people are thrown around by the whims of their dragons, rather than using their brains to plan their lives and follow through on their goals. Many dragons are happy to decide what you should do with your life.

### The One Page Miracle

To help you know what you want, I have developed an exercise called the One Page Miracle.[8] It is a powerful yet simple motivation exercise. It will help guide your thoughts, words, and actions. It is called the One Page Miracle because I've seen this exercise quickly focus and change many people's lives.

**Directions:** On a piece of paper, or on a digital form, clearly write out your major goals in the following areas. The areas of relationships, school, work, finances, and self are separated in order to encourage a more balanced

# MY ONE PAGE MIRACLE

*What Do I Want? What Am I Doing to Make It Happen?*

**RELATIONSHIPS**

SPOUSE/LOVE: _____

_____

_____

PARENTS: _____

_____

_____

CHILDREN: _____

_____

_____

FAMILY/FRIENDS: _____

_____

_____

NEIGHBORS: _____

_____

_____

WORK: _____

SCHOOL: _____

_____

_____

FINANCES: _____

_____

**SELF**

PHYSICAL HEALTH: _____

_____

EMOTIONAL HEALTH: _____

_____

SPIRITUAL HEALTH: _____

_____

approach to life. Burnout occurs when our lives become unbalanced and we overextend ourselves in one area while ignoring another.

**Relationships:** spouse/love, parents, children, family/friends, neighbors

**Work or School:** short- and long-term school and work goals

**Money:** short- and long-term financial goals

**Self:** physical, emotional, and spiritual health

In each section, succinctly write out what's important to you in that area; write what you want, not what you don't want. Be positive, use the first person, and include what you are currently doing to achieve these goals. With confidence and the expectation that you will make it happen, work on these goals over time. After you finish it, look at your One Page Miracle every day. Then before you do or say anything, ask yourself, *Is my behavior getting me what I want?*

If you focus on your goals every day, your brain receives and creates reality. When you give it some direction, it becomes much easier for you to match your behavior to get what you want. Your life becomes more intentional and less influenced by your dragons. Your Dragon Tamer starts to help you design your life.

Work toward goals that are important to you. Use the One Page Miracle to help you be the one who has the say. Once you know what you want, eliminate anything that hurts your Dragon Tamer and strengthen it with these strategies:

- Exercise to boost blood flow
- Learn new things to keep your brain active
- Supplement with omega-3 fatty acids and a multiple vitamin
- Optimize your vitamin D level with supplements or by getting more sun
- Protect your brain from trauma
- Avoid toxins, especially marijuana and alcohol
- Work to get to a healthy weight
- Make sleep a priority, targeting to get seven to eight hours each night
- Keep your blood sugar stable

You are more likely to be able to protect yourself from dragons and ANTs when you have clear goals, a healthy blood-sugar level, plenty of sleep, no alcohol in your system, and you are not hungry, angry, lonely, or tired. If you leave your PFC weak, you're more susceptible to Bad Habit Dragons, Scheming Dragons, and Addicted Dragons. When your Dragon Tamer is strong, you're the one in charge. And that's a powerful place to be.

---

*You are more likely to be able to protect yourself from dragons and ANTs when you have clear goals, a healthy blood-sugar level, plenty of sleep, no alcohol in your system, and you are not hungry, angry, lonely, or tired.*

---

# FINAL THOUGHTS

## REDIRECT WHAT YOUR BRAIN IS LISTENING TO, AND MAKE SURE OTHERS KNOW ABOUT THE DRAGONS

Brain health has been my passion for 40 years. Looking at the brain changed the way I practiced medicine and psychiatry, as well as the way I live my life. Now, over 175,000 brain scans later, it's become even more clear that the problems we treat aren't *mental health* issues; they're *brain health* issues that steal your mind. Enhancing biological brain health is a foundational aspect of how we help our patients get better, but it is only one piece of the wellness puzzle. Taming dragons is another piece of that puzzle. Helping people learn to keep their dragons in check is one of the keys to staying on the path to recovery from anxiety, depression, bad habits, and addictions. Because when life throws you for a loop—think of how the coronavirus pandemic has threatened our health, the health of our loved ones, our jobs, and our daily routines—it can unleash once-tamed dragons, allowing them to run wild again.

That's what happened to me when my father died after he had beaten COVID-19. I've been enhancing my brain health, teaching my patients how to tame their dragons, and helping them cope with death for decades. I know what I need to do, and yet, when faced with the loss of my dad combined with the added stresses of the pandemic, it had the potential to really get to me. I was vulnerable to the Grief, Loss, and Death Dragons interfering with my life. Yet I recognized them and followed the same strategies I have shared with you in this book to minimize their destructive ways. This doesn't mean that I'm not sad about losing my dad or that I'm no longer grieving. I am. But I'm not listening to my Dragons from the Past or allowing them to derail me from my brain-healthy habits or make me more vulnerable to the Scheming Dragons that want to hook me into bad habits and addictions. My Dragon Tamer (PFC) maintains control.

In your life, dragons will assault you every day. Some days they'll be whispering inside your head. Other days, when stress and anxiety are through the roof, they'll be screaming incessantly. Whether you listen to them depends on the health of your brain and the strength of your Dragon Tamer (your PFC). You'll know your dragons are running wild if they are impairing how you think, feel, or act. But if you've tamed them, they will help fuel you to achieve your purpose in life, even in the most distressing times.

For example, Sam, a longtime successful sports marketing entrepreneur, saw the entire professional sports industry come to a grinding halt during the pandemic and lost all his income for the foreseeable future. When he reached out to me for help in the first few weeks, he was anxious and angry that the business and identity he had worked so hard to achieve looked like it was dead in the water. During our session, he spent much of the time blaming others for his situation. His Dragons from the Past—the Anxious, Angry, and Judgmental ones—were breathing fire on his brain and impacting his actions. He was sinking into bad habits—drinking to soothe his anxiety, yelling at his family, and spending hours on social media railing against the forces he thought were behind the spread of the virus and shutdown restrictions. None of this was going to help him reach his goals to get his business back on track and feel like the smart, creative, accomplished man he had been.

We worked together on the strategies to tame his dragons and to enhance his brain health. Eventually he was able to turn himself around and stop dwelling on everything that was going wrong. He stopped looking for someone to blame and started taking responsibility for his life. He stopped blowing up at home over every little thing and started deep breathing or time-outs whenever he felt his frustration rising. He also stopped drinking to calm his anxious thoughts and purposely redirected his thinking to focus on laying the groundwork for a new business using the skills he had developed over the years. By the time the stay-at-home orders were lifting, he was already beginning to sign on new clients.

Learning how to tame your dragons will break your bad habits, reduce your vulnerability to schemers, shut down self-defeating thinking, and heal your addictions. That's powerful stuff. Redirect their energy to help you rather than hurt you. When you really start to hear what your brain is listening to, you will become much more cautious about what you allow to influence you and those you love. With enhanced emotional well-being, you'll feel more confident and resilient so you can face whatever life throws your way, whether it's a relationship breakup, an unexpected job layoff, or a pandemic.

What can be empowering is sharing what you've learned with others. By helping others tame their dragons, it's less likely that their dragons will try to pick a fight with yours. It creates more peace, more happiness, and better relationships in our society at large.

That's what Miley Cyrus did. After she discovered how to tame the Anxious, Hopeless, Helpless, and Grief and Loss Dragons that rose up within her when the coronavirus pandemic descended on the world, she turned around and showed her followers how they could take control of their own dragons. She helped create an army of Dragon Tamers who would continue to disseminate the word to outpace the fear that was spreading from COVID-19. Of course, not everybody has access to over 100 million followers like Miley does, but each of us has people we care about—our families, friends, coworkers, neighbors, fellow churchgoers, and social media networks. When you share with the people you care about—no matter how many or how few—you help create a growing legion of Dragon Tamers. So start today. Share what you've learned with someone you love.

# About Daniel G. Amen, MD

The *Washington Post* has called Dr. Amen the most popular psychiatrist in America, Sharecare named him the web's most influential expert and advocate on mental health, and he was the 2019 recipient of the John Maxwell Transformational Leadership Award.

Dr. Amen is a physician, double board-certified child, adolescent, and adult psychiatrist, 12-time *New York Times* bestselling author, and international speaker. He is the founder of Amen Clinics in Costa Mesa, Los Angeles, and San Francisco, California; Bellevue, Washington; Reston, Virginia; Atlanta, Georgia; New York, New York; Chicago, Illinois; and Dallas, Texas. Amen Clinics have one of the highest published success rates treating complex psychiatric issues, and they have built the world's largest database of functional brain scans, totaling more than 175,000 scans on patients from 155 countries.

Dr. Amen is the lead researcher on the world's largest brain imaging and rehabilitation study on professional football players. His research has not only demonstrated high levels of brain damage in players, but it also showed the possibility of significant recovery for many with the principles that underlie his work.

Together with Pastor Rick Warren and Mark Hyman, MD, Dr. Amen is also one of the chief architects of The Daniel Plan, a program to get the world healthy through religious organizations.

Dr. Amen is the author or coauthor of more than 80 professional articles, seven book chapters, and more than 30 books, including the #1 *New York Times* bestsellers *The Daniel Plan* and *Change Your Brain, Change Your Life*; as well as *The End of Mental Illness*; *Memory Rescue*; *Magnificent Mind at Any Age*; *Change Your Brain, Change Your Body*; *Use Your Brain to Change Your Age*; *Healing ADD*; *The Brain Warrior's Way*; and *The Brain Warrior's Way Cookbook*.

Dr. Amen's published scientific articles have appeared in the prestigious journals *Brain Imaging and Behavior*, Nature's *Molecular Psychiatry*, *PLOS ONE*, Nature's *Translational Psychiatry*, Nature's *Obesity*, *Journal of Neuropsychiatry and Clinical Neurosciences*, *Minerva Psichiatrica*,

*Journal of Neurotrauma, American Journal of Psychiatry, Nuclear Medicine Communications, Neurological Research, Journal of the American Academy of Child & Adolescent Psychiatry, Primary Psychiatry, Military Medicine,* and *General Hospital Psychiatry.* His research on post-traumatic stress disorder and traumatic brain injury was recognized by *Discover* magazine in its Year in Science issue as one of the "100 Top Stories of 2015."

Dr. Amen has written, produced, and hosted 15 popular shows about the brain on public television, which have aired more than 120,000 times across North America. He has appeared in movies, including *After the Last Round* and *The Crash Reel,* and in Emmy Award–winning television shows, such as *The Truth About Drinking, Dr. Phil,* and *The Dr. Oz Show.* He was a consultant on the movie *Concussion,* starring Will Smith. He has also spoken for the National Security Agency (NSA), the National Science Foundation (NSF), Harvard's Learning & the Brain Conference, the Department of the Interior, the National Council of Juvenile and Family Court Judges, and the Supreme Courts of Delaware, Ohio, and Wyoming. Dr. Amen's work has been featured in *Newsweek, Time* magazine, the *Huffington Post,* the BBC, the *Guardian, Parade* magazine, the *New York Times,* the *New York Times Magazine,* the *Washington Post,* the *Los Angeles Times, Men's Health,* and *Cosmopolitan.*

Dr. Amen is married to Tana. He is the father of four children and grandfather to Elias, Emmy, Liam, Louie, and Haven. He is an avid table tennis player.

# Gratitude and Appreciation

So many people have been involved in the process of creating *Your Brain Is Always Listening*. I am grateful to them all, especially the tens of thousands of patients and families who have come to Amen Clinics and allowed us to help them on their healing journey.

I am grateful to the amazing staff at Amen Clinics, who work hard every day serving our patients. Special appreciation to Frances Sharpe who helped me craft the book to make it accessible to our readers. Also, to my friends and colleagues Dr. Sharon May (who initially taught me about the dragons), Dr. Rob Johnson, Kim Schneider, Tom and Christine Bowen, Michelle Walthall, Christine Perkins, Rob Patterson, Jim Springer, and Natalie Buchoz for their input, love, and support. I am also grateful to Jan Long Harris and the team at Tyndale for their belief in the book and help in getting it to the world, and to my editor, Andrea Vinley Converse, who helped make this book the best it can be.

I am grateful to my amazing wife, Tana, who is my partner in all I do, and to my family, who have tolerated my obsession with making brains better. Special thanks to our daughter Chloe and our nieces Amelie and Alizé, who listened endlessly to my talking about the dragons. I love you all.

# Resources

## AMEN CLINICS

amenclinics.com

Amen Clinics, Inc. (ACI), was established in 1989 by Daniel G. Amen, MD. We specialize in innovative diagnosis and treatment planning for a wide variety of behavioral, learning, emotional, cognitive, and weight issues for children, teenagers, and adults. ACI has an international reputation for evaluating brain-behavior problems, such as ADD/ADHD, depression, anxiety, school failure, traumatic brain injury and concussions, obsessive- compulsive disorders, aggressiveness, marital conflict, cognitive decline, brain toxicity from drugs or alcohol, and obesity. In addition, we work with people to optimize brain function and decrease the risk for Alzheimer's disease and other age-related issues.

Brain SPECT imaging is one of the primary diagnostic tools used in our clinics. ACI has the world's largest database of brain scans for emotional, cognitive, and behavioral problems. ACI welcomes referrals from physicians, psychologists, social workers, marriage and family therapists, drug and alcohol counselors, and individual patients and families.

Our toll-free number is (888) 564-2700.

Amen Clinics Orange County,
California
3150 Bristol St., Suite 400
Costa Mesa, CA 92626

Amen Clinics Northern California
350 N. Wiget Ln., Suite 105
Walnut Creek, CA 94598

Amen Clinics Northwest
616 120th Ave. NE, Suite C100
Bellevue, WA 98005

Amen Clinics Los Angeles
5363 Balboa Blvd., Suite 100
Encino, CA 91316

Amen Clinics Washington, D.C.
1875 Campus Commons Dr.
Reston, VA 20191

Amen Clinics New York
16 East 40th St., 9th Floor
New York, NY 10016

Amen Clinics Atlanta
5901-C Peachtree Dunwoody
Road, N.E., Suite 65
Atlanta, GA 30328

Amen Clinics Chicago
2333 Waukegan Rd., Suite 100
Bannockburn, IL 60015

Amen Clinics Dallas
7301 N. State Hwy 161, Suite 170
Irving, TX 75039

Our website, amenclinics.com, is educational and interactive, geared toward mental health and medical professionals, educators, students, and the public. It contains a wealth of information and resources to help you learn about optimizing your brain. The site contains more than 300 color brain SPECT images, thousands of scientific abstracts on brain SPECT imaging for psychiatry, a free brain health assessment, and much, much more.

## BRAIN FIT LIFE

*mybrainfitlife.com*

Based on Dr. Amen's 35 years as a clinical psychiatrist, he and his wife, Tana, have developed a sophisticated online community to help you feel smarter, happier, and younger. It includes:

- Detailed questionnaires to help you know your brain type and a personalized program targeted to your own needs
- WebNeuro, a sophisticated neuropsychological test that assesses your brain
- Fun brain games and tools to boost your motivation
- Exclusive, award-winning, 24-7 brain gym membership
- Physical exercises and tutorials led by Tana
- Hundreds of Tana's delicious, brain-healthy recipes
- Exercises to kill the ANTs (automatic negative thoughts)
- Meditation and hypnosis audios for sleep, anxiety, peak performance, and overcoming pain and weight issues

- Amazing brain-enhancing music by Grammy Award-winner Barry Goldstein
- Online forum for questions and answers and a community of support
- Access to monthly live coaching calls with Daniel and Tana

## BRAINMD

*brainmd.com*

For the highest-quality brain health supplements, courses, books, and information products

# Notes

## INTRODUCTION: YOUR BRAIN IS ALWAYS LISTENING TO HIDDEN DRAGONS

1. "Dr. Amen: Episode 1," *Bright Minded: Live with Miley Cyrus,* March 17, 2020, https://www.youtube.com/watch?v=LZaJJWCpLWc.

2. Keith Sharon, "Elderly O.C. Couple Recovers from Coronavirus, Swears by Hydroxychloroquine," *Orange County Register*, April 16, 2020, https://www.ocregister .com/2020/04/16/coronavirus-elderly-oc-couple-recovers-swears-by-controversial -treatment/.

3. Centers for Disease Control and Prevention, "Severe Outcomes among Patients with Coronavirus Disease 2019 (COVID-19)—United States, February 12–March 16, 2020," *Morbidity and Mortality Weekly Report* 69, no.12 (March 27, 2020): 343–346, https://cdc .gov/mmwr/volumes/69/wr/mm6912e2.htm.

## YOUR BRAIN: A VERY BRIEF PRIMER

1. Majid Fotuhi, "Can You Grow Your Hippocampus? Yes. Here's How, and Why It Matters," SharpBrains, November 4, 2015, https://sharpbrains.com/blog/2015/11/04/can-you -grow-your-hippocampus-yes-heres-how-and-why-it-matters/.

2. Daniel Amen, *Change Your Brain, Change Your Life*, rev. ed., (New York: Harmony Books, 2015), 44, 49–55.

3. Read more about the BRIGHT MINDS risk factors in *Memory Rescue* or *The End of Mental Illness*.

## SECTION 1: TAME THE DRAGONS FROM THE PAST

1. "A Neuropsychiatrist Explains Why Kobe's Death Hurts Us So Much," Amen Clinics, January 30, 2020, https://www.amenclinics.com/blog/a-neuropsychiatrist-explains-why -kobes-death-hurts-us-so-much/.

2. Adam Leipzig, "How to Know Your Life Purpose in 5 Minutes," TEDx Malibu, video, 10:33, February 1, 2013, https://www.youtube.com/watch?v=vVsXO9brK7M&list=PLiKtxxcS-pbQ 9BPH68bS6yPK1L7T4GmLW&index=5.

3. Michelle C. Carlson et al., "Impact of the Baltimore Experience Corps Trial on Cortical and Hippocampal Volumes," *Alzheimers & Dementia* 11, no.11 (November 2015): 1340–1348.

4. Susie Moore, "7 Things to Remember When Feeling Inferior," *Huff Post*, February 4, 2016, https://huffpost.com/entry/7-things-to-remember-when-feeling-inferior_b_9142320.

5. "Any Anxiety Disorder," National Institute of Mental Health, updated November 2017, https://www.nimh.nih.gov/health/statistics/any-anxiety-disorder.shtml.

6. "America's State of Mind Report," Express Scripts, April 16, 2020, https://www.express -scripts.com/corporate/americas-state-of-mind-report.

7. "Keys to Long Life? Not What You Might Expect," *Science Daily*, March 12, 2011, https://www.sciencedaily.com/releases/2011/03/110311153541.htm.

8. Peter Boelens et al., "A Randomized Trial of the Effect of Prayer on Depression and Anxiety," *International Journal of Psychiatry in Medicine* 39, no.4 (2009): 377–392, https://pubmed.ncbi.nlm.nih.gov/20391859/.

9. Xianglong Zeng et al., "The Effect of Loving-Kindness Meditation on Positive Emotions: A Meta-Analytic Review," *Frontiers in Psychology* 6, (November 3, 2015): 1693.

   Barbara L. Fredrickson et al., "Open Hearts Build Lives: Positive Emotions, Induced through Loving-Kindness Meditation, Build Consequential Personal Resources," *Journal of Personality and Social Psychology* 95, no.5 (November 2008): 1045–1062.

10. James W. Carson et al., "Loving-Kindness Meditation for Chronic Low Back Pain: Results from a Pilot Trial," *Journal of Holistic Nursing* 23, no.3 (September 2005): 287–304.

11. Makenzie E. Tonelli and Amy B. Wachholtz, "Meditation-Based Treatment Yielding Immediate Relief for Meditation-Naïve Migraineurs," *Pain Management Nursing* 15, no.1 (March 2014): 36–40.

12. David J. Kearney et al., "Loving-Kindness Meditation for Posttraumatic Stress Disorder: A Pilot Study," *Journal of Traumatic Stress* 26, no. 4 (August 2013): 426–434.

13. Alexander J. Stell and Tom Farsides, "Brief Loving-Kindness Meditation Reduces Racial Bias, Mediated by Positive Other-Regarding Emotions," *Motivation and Emotion* 40, no.1 (September 9, 2015): 140–147.

14. Mei-Kei Leung et al., "Increased Gray Matter Volume in the Right Angular and Posterior Parahippocampal Gyri in Loving-Kindness Meditators," *Social Cognitive and Affective Neuroscience* 8, no. 1 (January 2013): 34–39.

15. Bethany E. Kok et al., "How Positive Emotions Build Physical Health: Perceived Positive Social Connections Account for the Upward Spiral between Positive Emotions and Vagal Tone," *Psychological Science* 24, no.7 (July 2013): 1123–1132.

16. Sarah C. P. Williams, "Study Identifies Brain Areas Altered during Hypnotic Trances," press release, Stanford School of Medicine, July 28, 2016, https://med.stanford.edu /news/all-news/2016/07/study-identifies-brain-areas-altered-during-hypnotic-trances .html#:~:text=Brain%20activity%20and%20connectivity,of%20the%20brain%20 under%20hypnosis.&text=%E2%80%9CIn%20hypnosis%2C%20you're,control%20 perception%20and%20our%20bodies.

   Heidi Jiang et al., "Brain Activity and Functional Connectivity Associated with Hypnosis," *Cerebral Cortex* 27, no.8 (August 2017): 4083–4093.

17. Psychiatrist Judith Cohen and psychologists Anthony Mannarino and Esther Deblinger developed TF-CBT.

18. Nicolas Gwozdziewycz and Lewis Mehl-Madrona, "Meta-Analysis of the Use of Narrative Exposure Therapy for the Effects of Trauma Among Refugee Populations," *The Permanente Journal* 17, no. 1 (Winter 2013): 70–76, https://www.ncbi.nlm.nih.gov/pmc /articles/PMC3627789/.

19. Amy S. Leiner et al., "Avoidant Coping and Treatment Outcome in Rape-Related Posttraumatic Stress Disorder," *Journal of Consulting and Clinical Psychology* 80, no. 2 (April 2012): 317–321, https://content.apa.org/record/2012-00396-001.

20. Amanda J. Shallcross et al., "Let It Be: Accepting Negative Emotional Experiences Predicts Decreased Negative Affect and Depressive Symptoms," *Behaviour Research and Therapy* 48, no. 9 (September 2010): 921–929, https://www.ncbi.nlm.nih.gov/pmc /articles/PMC3045747/.

21. Luana Marques et al., "A Comparison of Emotional Approach Coping (EAC) between Individuals with Anxiety Disorders and Nonanxious Controls," *CNS Neuroscience & Therapeutics* 15, no. 2 (June 2009): 100–106.

22. Daniel G. Amen, *Feel Better Fast and Make It Last* (Carol Stream, IL: Tyndale Momentum, 2018), 152–153.

23. Karen Lansing et al., "High-Resolution Brain SPECT Imaging and Eye Movement Desensitization and Reprocessing in Police Officers with PTSD," *Journal of Neuropsychiatry and Clinical Neurosciences* 17, no. 4 (Fall 2005): 526–532.

24. Brian Mullen et al., "Exploring the Safety and Therapeutic Effects of Deep Pressure Stimulation Using a Weighted Blanket," *Occupational Therapy in Mental Health* 24, no. 1 (March 2008): 65–89.

25. Hannah Frishberg, "Doing Good Deeds Actually Reduces Physical Pain: Study," *New York Post*, December 31, 2019, https://nypost.com/2019/12/31/doing-good-deeds-actually -reduces-physical-pain-study/?utm_campaign=iosapp&utm_source=mail_app.

26. John Townsend, *People Fuel: Fill Your Tank for Life, Love, and Leadership* (Grand Rapids, MI: Zondervan, 2019).

27. Jennifer S. Lerner et al., "Effects of Fear and Anger on Perceived Risks of Terrorism: A National Field Experiment," *Psychological Science* 14, no. 2 (March 2003): 144–150.

28. Everett Worthington, "Research," accessed on June 29, 2020, http://www.evworthington -forgiveness.com/research.

29. Kirsten Weir, "Forgiveness Can Improve Mental and Physical Health. Research Shows How to Get There," *Monitor on Psychology* 48, no. 1 (January 2017): 31–33, https://www.apa.org/monitor/2017/01/ce-corner.

30. Sarah Corker, "Has the Virus Prompted an Early Mid-Life Crisis for Some?" BBC News, May 24, 2020, https://bbc.com/news/business-5275540.

31. Elisabeth Kübler-Ross, *Death: The Final Stage of Growth* (New York: Touchstone, 1975), 164.

32. Mehrdad Kalantari et al., "Efficacy of Writing for Recovery on Traumatic Grief Symptoms of Afghani Refugee Bereaved Adolescents: A Randomized Control Trial," *Omega* 65, no. 2 (October 2012): 139–150.

33. Karolijne van der Houwen et al., "The Efficacy of a Brief Internet-Based Self-Help Intervention for the Bereaved," *Behaviour Research and Therapy* 48, no. 5 (May 2010): 359–367.

34. Lillian M. Range et al., "Does Writing about the Bereavement Lessen Grief Following Sudden, Unintentional Death?" *Death Studies* 24, no. 2 (March 2000): 115–134.

35. Marilyn A. Mendoza, "When Grief Gets Physical," *Psychology Today*, September 4, 2019, https://www.psychologytoday.com/us/blog/understanding-grief/201909/when-grief-gets -physical.

36. Illumeably, "What a Psychiatrist Learned from 87,000 Brain Scans," Illumeably, November 13, 2017, video, 6:57, https://www.facebook.com/watch/?v=283984572006650/.

37. Martin E. P. Seligman et al., "Positive Psychology Progress: Empirical Validation of Interventions," *American Psychologist* 60, no. 5 (July–August 2005): 410–421.

38. Karin Rippstein-Leuenberger et al., "A Qualitative Analysis of the Three Good Things Intervention in Healthcare Workers," *BMJ Open* 7, no. 5 (June 13, 2017): e015826.

39. "Hans Selye Quotes and Sayings—Page 1," Inspiring Quotes, 2020, https://www. inspiringquotes.us/author/9982-hans-selye.

40. Tristen K. Inagaki et al., "The Neurobiology of Giving Versus Receiving Support: The Role of Stress-Related and Social Reward-Related Neural Activity," *Psychosomatic Medicine* 78, no. 4 (May 2016): 443–453.

41. Albert Bender, "Suicide Sweeping Indian Country Is Genocide," *People's World*, May 18, 2015, https://www.peoplesworld.org/article/suicide-sweeping-indian-country-is -genocide/.

42. David Pagliaccio et al., "Brain Volume Abnormalities in Youth at High Risk for Depression: Adolescent Brain and Cognitive Development Study," *Journal of the American Academy of Child & Adolescent Psychiatry* (October 18, 2019): https://doi.org/10.1016/j .jaac.2019.09.032.

43. Sandro Galea, Raina M. Merchant, and Nicole Lurie, "The Mental Health Consequences of COVID-19 and Physical Distancing: The Need for Prevention and Early Intervention" *JAMA Internal Medicine* 180, no. 6 (April 10, 2020): 817–818, https://jamanetwork .com/journals/jamainternalmedicine/fullarticle/2764404.

44. "Prince William: Parenthood Brought Diana Death Emotions," BBC News, May 24, 2020, https://www.bbc.com/news/uk-52786833.

45. *The Curious Case of Benjamin Button*, directed by David Fincher (Hollywood, CA: Paramount, 2008).

## SECTION 2: QUIET THE THEY, THEM, AND OTHER DRAGONS

1. Byron Katie, Twitter, January 6, 2014, https://twitter.com/byronkatie/status/420234784640876544.

2. Karin Lehnardt, "62 Interesting Birth Order Facts," Fact Retriever, February 22, 2017, www.factretriever.com/birth-order-facts.

   Sandra E. Black, "New Evidence on the Impacts of Birth Order," National Bureau of Economic Research, accessed on June 30, 2020, http://data.nber.org/reporter/2017number4/black.html.

3. Marco Bertoni and Giorgio Brunello, "Later-Borns Don't Give Up: The Temporary Effects of Birth Order on European Earnings," *Demography* 53, no. 2 (April 2016): 449–470.

4. John M. Curtis and Donald R. Cowell, "Relation of Birth Order and Scores on Measures of Pathological Narcissism," *Psychological Reports* 72, no. 1 (February 1993): 311–315.

5. Rachel Hosie, "First-Borns Are the Worst Drivers, Finds Study," *Independent*, August 10, 2017, https://www.independent.co.uk/life-style/worst-drivers-first-born-children-siblings-cars-study-eldest-a7885496.html.

6. John Lim, "9 Scientific Facts That Make You Wish You Were the Middle Child," Says.com, http://says.com/my/fun/middle-children-are-the-coolest.

7. I first shared this story in *Change Your Brain, Change Your Life*, rev. ed. (New York: Harmony Books, 2015), 116.

8. Kieron Barclay et al., "Birth Order and Hospitalization for Alcohol and Narcotics Use in Sweden," *Drug and Alcohol Dependence* 167 (October 1, 2016): 15–22.

9. Christa Spraggins, "The Only Child: Everything You Need to Know, Answered by Research," *Research Addict*, December 9, 2018, https://researchaddict.com/only-child-effects/.

10. Emine Saner, "The Truth about Only Children: Are They More Insular and Confident?" *Guardian*, May 31, 2018, https://www.theguardian.com/lifeandstyle/2018/may/31/truth-about-only-children-insular-confident-worry.

    Anushka Asthana. "An Only Child is a Happy Child, Says Research," *Guardian*, November 13, 2010,https://www.theguardian.com/lifeandstyle/2010/nov/14/only-children-happier-competition-bullying.

    Yehui Lao et al. "The Only Child, Birth Order and Educational Outcomes," Economics Discussion Papers, No. 2019-7, 2019, Kiel Institute for the World Economy. http://www.economics-ejournal.org/economics/discussionpapers/2019-7.

11. Joshua K. Hartshorne, "How Birth Order Affects Your Personality," *Scientific American Mind*, January 1, 2010, https://www.scientificamerican.com/article/ruled-by-birth-order/.

12. Arthur Aron et al., "Reward, Motivation, and Emotion Systems Associated with Early-Stage Intense Romantic Love," *Journal of Neurophysiology* 94, no. 1 (July 2005): 327–337.

13. Helen E. Fisher et al., "Intense, Passionate, Romantic Love: A Natural Addiction? How the Fields That Investigate Romance and Substance Abuse Can Inform Each Other," *Frontiers in Psychology* 7 (May 10, 2016): 687.

## SECTION 3: TAME THE THOUGHTS THAT FUEL YOUR DRAGONS

1. Natalie L. Marchant et al., "Repetitive Negative Thinking Is Associated with Amyloid, Tau, and Cognitive Decline," *Alzheimer's & Dementia* 16, no. 7 (June 7, 2020): 1054–1064, https://alz-journals.onlinelibrary.wiley.com/doi/full/10.1002/alz.12116.

2. Daniel G. Amen, *Change Your Brain, Change Your Life*, rev. ed. (New York: Harmony Books, 2015), 109–117.

3. Amen, *Change Your Brain, Change Your Life*, 114.

4. Byron Katie, *Loving What Is: Four Questions That Can Change Your Life* (New York: Harmony Books, 2002).

## SECTION 4: ELIMINATE BAD HABIT DRAGONS

1. James Clear, *Atomic Habits* (New York: Avery, 2018).
2. Bella M. DePaulo et al., "Lying in Everyday Life," *Journal of Personality and Social Psychology* 70, no. 5 (June 1996): 979–995.
3. Andrea Gurmankin Levy et al., "Prevalence of and Factors Associated with Patient Nondisclosure of Medically Relevant Information to Clinicians," *JAMA Network Open* 1, no. 7 (November 2, 2018): e185293.
4. "Landmark Report: U.S. Teens Use an Average of Nine Hours of Media Per Day, Tweens Use Six Hours: New 'Media Use Census' from Common Sense Details Media Habits and Preferences of American 8- to 18-Year-Olds," Common Sense Media, November 3, 2015, https://www.commonsensemedia.org/about-us/news/press-releases/landmark-report -us-teens-use-an-average-of-nine-hours-of-media-per-day.
5. James B. Weaver et al., "Health-Risk Correlates of Video-Game Playing among Adults," *American Journal of Preventive Medicine* 37, no. 4 (October 2009): 299–305.
6. Ian Bogost, "The Cigarette of This Century," *Atlantic*, June 6, 2012, https://www.theatlantic .com/technology/archive/2012/06/the-cigarette-of-this-century/258092/.
7. Kevin McSpadden, "You Now Have a Shorter Attention Span Than a Goldfish," *Time*, May 14, 2015, https://time.com/3858309/attention-spans-goldfish/.
8. James Clear, *Atomic Habits* (New York: Avery, 2018).
9. Heike Bruch and Sumantra Ghoshal, "Beware the Busy Manager," *Harvard Business Review*, February 2002, https://hbr.org/2002/02/beware-the-busy-manager.
10. Yaser Ghanam, "Why Agile Methods Work," InfoQ, December 12, 2012, https://www.infoq .com/articles/why-agile-methods-work/.
11. Daniel G. Amen, *Healing ADD*, rev. ed. (New York: Berkley, 2013), chapter 16.
12. National Center for Health Statistics, "Obesity and Overweight," Centers for Disease Control and Prevention, June 13, 2016, http://www.cdc.gov/nchs/fastats/obesity -overweight.htm.
13. Thomas Spoehr and Bridget Handy, "The Looming National Security Crisis: Young Americans Unable to Serve in the Military," The Heritage Foundation, February 18, 2018, https://www.heritage.org/defense/report/the-looming-national-security-crisis-young -americans-unable-serve-the-military.
14. Craig M. Hales et al. "Prevalence of Obesity Among Adults and Youth: United States 2015–2016," NCHS Data Brief, no. 288, October 2017, https://www.cdc.gov/nchs/data /databriefs/db288.pdf.
15. Daniel G. Amen and Tana Amen, *The Brain Warrior's Way* (New York: New American Library, 2016), 40, 42–43.
16. "The Power of Prevention: Chronic Disease . . . the Public Health Challenge of the 21st Century," National Center for Chronic Disease Prevention and Health Promotion, 2009, https://www.cdc.gov/chronicdisease/pdf/2009-Power-of-Prevention.pdf.

## SECTION 5: OUTFOX THE SCHEMING DRAGONS

1. Nir Eyal, *Hooked: How to Build Habit-Forming Products* (New York: Portfolio/Penguin, 2014).
2. Susan Weinschenk, "Use Unpredictable Rewards to Keep Behavior Going," *Psychology Today*, November 13, 2013, https://www.psychologytoday.com/us/blog/brain -wise/201311/use-unpredictable-rewards-keep-behavior-going.
3. W. Spencer Murch et al., "Measuring the Slot Machine Zone with Attentional Dual Tasks and Respiratory Sinus Arrhythmia," *Psychology of Addictive Behaviors* 31, no. 3 (May 2017): 375–384.
4. "Kids Meals, Toys, and TV Advertising: A Triple Threat to Child Health," *Journal of Pediatrics*, news release, October 30, 2015, http://www.jpeds.com/content/JPEDSEmond.

5. Read more about the strategies of food corporations in *The Brain Warrior's Way* (New York: New American Library, 2016), 44–52.

6. M. Shahbandeh, "Retail Value of Health and Wellness Products in North America in 2017, by Country (in Billion U.S. Dollars)," Statista, October 8, 2018, http://statista.com/statistics/888018/retail-sales-of-health-and-wellness-products-in-north-america-by-country/.

7. Research and Markets, "United States Weight Loss and Diet Control Market Report 2019: 2018 Results and 2019–2023 Forecasts—Top Competitors Ranking with 30-Year Revenue Analysis," PR Newswire, February 27, 2019, https://www.prnewswire.com/news-releases/united-states-weight-loss--diet-control-market-report-2019-2018-results--2019-2023-forecasts---top-competitors-ranking-with-30-year-revenue-analysis-300803186.html.

8. Steven H. Woolf and Laudan Aron, eds., "U.S. Health in International Perspective: Shorter Lives, Poorer Health," (Washington, DC: The National Academies Press, 2013), https://www.nap.edu/read/13497/chapter/1.

9. Alicia Rubin, "Marijuana Sales Spike During COVID-19 Pandemic," KDRV.com, April 20, 2020, https://www.kdrv.com/content/news/Marijuana-sales-spike-during-COVID-19-pandemic-569803561.html.

10. Daniel G. Amen et al., "Discriminative Properties of Hippocampal Hypoperfusion in Marijuana Users Compared to Healthy Controls: Implications for Marijuana Administration in Alzheimer's Dementia," *Journal of Alzheimer's Disease* 56, no. 1 (2017): 261–273.

11. Daniel G. Amen et al., "Patterns of Regional Cerebral Blood Flow as a Function of Age throughout the Lifespan," *Journal of Alzheimer's Disease* 65, no. 4 (2018): 1087–1092, https://pubmed.ncbi.nlm.nih.gov/30103336/.

12. Roni Caryn Rabin, "Federal Agency Courted Alcohol Industry to Fund Study on Benefits of Moderate Drinking," *New York Times*, March 17, 2018, https://www.nytimes.com/2018/03/17/health/nih-alcohol-study-liquor-industry.html.

13. "Alcohol Use and Cancer," American Cancer Society, June 9, 2020, https://www.cancer.org/cancer/cancer-causes/diet-physical-activity/alcohol-use-and-cancer.html.

14. American Cancer Society, "American Cancer Society Updates Diet and Physical Activity Guideline for Cancer Prevention," press release, June 9, 2020, https://pressroom.cancer.org/DietPhysicalActivity2020.

15. Caitlin Dewey, "'Quarantinis' and Beer Chugs: Is the Pandemic Driving Us to Drink?" *Guardian*, April 27, 2020, https://www.theguardian.com/us-news/2020/apr/27/coronavirus-pandemic-drinking-alcohol.

16. "E-cigarettes: Facts, Stats and Regulations," Truth Initiative, November 11, 2019, https://truthinitiative.org/research-resources/emerging-tobacco-products/e-cigarettes-facts-stats-and-regulations.

17. "Teens Using Vaping Devices in Record Numbers," December 17, 2018, National Institute on Drug Abuse, https://www.drugabuse.gov/news-events/news-releases/2018/12/teens-using-vaping-devices-in-record-numbers.

18. "E-cigarettes: Facts, Stats and Regulations," Truth Initiative, November 11, 2019, https://truthinitiative.org/research-resources/emerging-tobacco-products/e-cigarettes-facts-stats-and-regulations.

19. "America's State of Mind Report," Express Scripts, April 16, 2020, https://www.express-scripts.com/corporate/americas-state-of-mind-report.

20. Erika Edwards, "Antidepressant Zoloft and Generic Version in Short Supply, FDA Says," NBC News, June 3, 2020, nbcnews.com/health/health-news/antidepressant-zoloft-generic-version-short-supply-fda-says-n1223356.

21. "Lead in Lipstick," Campaign for Safe Cosmetics, 2020, www.safecosmetics.org/get-the-facts/regulations/us-laws/lead-in-lipstick/.

22. "Advertising Spending in the Perfumes, Cosmetics, and Other Toilet Preparations

Industry in the United States from 2018 to 2020 (in Million U.S. Dollars)," Statista, September 3, 2019, https://www.statista.com/statistics/470467/perfumes-cosmetics-and-other-toilet-preparations-industry-ad-spend-usa/.

23. Tanjaniina Laukkanen et al., "Sauna Bathing Is Inversely Associated with Dementia and Alzheimer's Disease in Middle-Aged Finnish Men," *Age and Ageing* 46, no. 2 (March 1, 2017): 245–249, https://academic.oup.com/ageing/article/46/2/245/2654230.

24. Aric Jenkins, "Netflix Earnings: 16 Million New Subscribers, Amid Pandemic," *Fortune*, April 21, 2020, https://fortune.com/2020/04/21/netflix-earnings-16-million-new-subscribers-despite-pandemic/.

25. Joan E. Solsman, "Disney Plus Has More Than 10 Million Subscribers," CNET, November 13, 2019, https://www.cnet.com/news/disney-plus-more-than-10-million-people-signed-up/.

26. Kenji Kobayashi and Ming Hsu, "Common Neural Code for Reward and Information Value," *Proceedings of the National Academy of Sciences of the United States of America* 116, no. 26 (June 25, 2019):13061–13066, https://doi.org/10.1073/pnas.1820145116.

27. Associated Press, "News Programs See Ratings Soar during Coronavirus Pandemic," *MarketWatch*, March 25, 2020, https://www.marketwatch.com/story/news-programs-see-ratings-soar-during-coronavirus-pandemic-2020-03-25.

28. "Study Finds Lure of Entertainment, Work Hard for People to Resist," UChicago News, January 27, 2012, https://news.uchicago.edu/story/study-finds-lure-entertainment-work-hard-people-resist.

29. Stephan Hamann et al., "Men and Women Differ in Amygdala Response to Visual Sexual Stimuli," *Nature Neuroscience* 7, (March 7, 2004): 411–416, https://www.nature.com/articles/nn1208.

30. Mark Regnerus et al., "Documenting Pornography Use in America: A Comparative Analysis of Methodological Approaches," *Journal of Sex Research* 53, no. 7 (December 18, 2015): 873–881, https://www.tandfonline.com/doi/abs/10.1080/00224499.2015.1096886.

31. Todd Love et al., "Neuroscience of Internet Pornography Addiction: A Review and Update," *Behavioral Sciences* (Basel, Switzerland) 5, no. 3 (September 2015): 388–433, https://www.ncbi.nlm.nih.gov/pmc/articles/PMC4600144/.

32. American Psychological Association, "APA *Stress in America* Survey: US at 'Lowest Point We Can Remember;' Future of Nation Most Commonly Reported Source of Stress," press release, November 1, 2017, https://www.apa.org/news/press/releases/2017/11/lowest-point.

33. Daria J. Kuss et al., "Neurobiological Correlates in Internet Gaming Disorder: A Systematic Literature Review," *Frontiers in Psychiatry* 9 (May 8, 2018): 166, https://www.frontiersin.org/articles/10.3389/fpsyt.2018.00166/full.

34. Ethan Kross et al., "Facebook Use Predicts Declines in Subjective Well-Being in Young Adults," *PLOS ONE* 8, no. 8 (August 14, 2013): e69841, https://journals.plos.org/plosone/article?id=10.1371/journal.pone.0069841.

35. Kevin Punsky, "Evidence Suggests Amateur Contact Sports Increase Risk of Degenerative Disorder," Mayo Clinic News Network, December 2, 2015, https://newsnetwork.mayoclinic.org/discussion/mayo-clinic-cte-fl-release/.

36. Greg Bishop, "When Helmet Safety Meets Capitalism," *Sports Illustrated*, November 20, 2019, https://www.si.com/nfl/2019/11/20/nfl-concussions-helmet-safety.

37. Adrian D. Garcia, "Survey: Holidays Bring Spending Stress for Most Americans," Bankrate, November 13, 2019, https://www.bankrate.com/surveys/holiday-gifting-november-2019/.

## SECTION 6: ADDICTED DRAGON RECOVERY PROGRAM

1. The 12 Steps are taken from *Alcoholics Anonymous: The Story of How Many Thousands of Men and Women Have Recovered from Alcoholism*, 2nd ed. (New York: Alcoholics

Anonymous World Services, 1955), 59–60. Comments in parentheses are from the author.

2. Lee Ann Kaskutas, "Alcoholics Anonymous Effectiveness: Faith Meets Science," *Journal of Addictive Diseases* 28,no. 2 (2009): 145–157.

3. Franklin Covey.com, "Habit 2: Begin with the End in Mind," https://www.franklincovey.com/the-7-habits/habit-2.html.

4. Kirsten Weir, "Forgiveness Can Improve Mental and Physical Health: Research Shows How to Get There," *Monitor on Psychology* 48, no. 1 (January 2017): 30, https://www.apa.org/monitor/2017/01/ce-corner.aspx.

5. I also wrote about brain types in *The Brain Warrior's Way* (New York: New American Library, 2016), 65–69.

6. S. Hirayama et al., "The Effect of Phosphatidylserine Administration on Memory and Symptoms of Attention-Deficit Hyperactivity Disorder: A Randomised, Double-Blind, Placebo-Controlled Clinical Trial," *Journal of Human Nutrition and Dietetics* 27, Suppl. 2 (April 2014): 284–291,https://doi: 10.1016/j.eurpsy.2011.05.004.

7. Purushottam Jangid et al., "Comparative Study of Efficacy of L-5-hydroxytryptophan and Fluoxetine in Patients Presenting with First Depressive Episode," *Asian Journal of Psychiatry* 6, no. 1 (February 2013): 29–34, https://www.sciencedirect.com/science/article/abs/pii/S1876201812001177?via%3Dihub.

Jules Angst, et al., "The Treatment of Depression with L-5-Hydroxytryptophan versus Imipramine. Results of Two Open and One Double-Blind Study," *Archiv für Psychiatrie und Nervenkrankheiten* (Berlin, Germany) 224, no. 2, (October 11, 1977):175–186.

8. "5-HTP," Examine.com, 2020, https://examine.com/supplements/5-htp/.

9. "Saffron," Examine.com, 2020, https;//examine.com/supplements/saffron/.

Adrian L. Lopresti and Peter D. Drummond, "Saffron (Crocus Sativus) for Depression: A Systematic Review of Clinical Studies and Examination of Underlying Antidepressant Mechanisms of Action," *Human Psychopharmacology* 29, no. 6 (November 2014): 517–527.

10. Magda Tsolaki et al., "Efficacy and Safety of Crocus Sativus L. in Patients with Mild Cognitive Impairment: One Year Single-Blind Randomized, with Parallel Groups, Clinical Trial," *Journal of Alzheimer's Disease* 54, no. 1 (July 27, 2016): 129–133, https://www.j-alz.com/content/efficacy-and-safety-crocus-sativus-patients-mild-cognitive-impairment.

11. Ladan Kashani et al., "Saffron for Treatment of Fluoxetine-Induced Sexual Dysfunction in Women: Randomized Double-Blind Placebo Controlled Study," *Human Psychopharmacology* 28, no. 1 (January 2013): 54–60.

12. Teodoro Bottiglieri, "S-Adenosyl-L-Methionine (SAMe): From the Bench to the Bedside— Molecular Basis of a Pleiotrophic Molecule," *American Journal of Clinical Nutrition* 76, no. 5 (November 2002): 1151S–1157S.

13. Anup Sharma et al., "S-Adenosylmethionine (SAMe) for Neuropsychiatric Disorders: A Clinician-Oriented Review of Research," *Journal of Clinical Psychiatry* 78, no. 6 (June 2017): e656–e667, https://www.psychiatrist.com/JCP/article/Pages/2017/v78n06/v78n0606.aspx.

14. Daniel G. Amen, *Memory Rescue* (Carol Stream, IL: Tyndale, 2017), 101.

15. R. Jorde et al., "Effects of Vitamin D Supplementation on Symptoms of Depression in Overweight and Obese Subjects: Randomized Double Blind Trial," *Journal of Internal Medicine* 264, no. 6 (December 2008): 599–609, https://pubmed.ncbi.nlm.nih.gov/18793245/.

16. Kate Janse Van Rensburg et al., "Acute Exercise Modulates Cigarette Cravings and Brain Activation in Response to Smoking-Related Images: An fMRI Study," *Psychopharmacology* 203, no. 3 (November 18, 2008): 589–598, https://link.springer.com/article/10.1007/s00213-008-1405-3.

17. Rachel L. Tomko et al., "N-Acetylcysteine: A Potential Treatment for Substance Use Disorders," *Current Psychiatry* 17, no. 6 (June 2018): 30–55, https://www.ncbi.nlm.nih.gov/pmc/articles/PMC5993450/.

18. Jon E Grant, Suck Won Kim, and Brian L. Odlaug, "N-Acetyl Cysteine, a Glutamate-Modulating Agent, in the Treatment of Pathological Gambling: A Pilot Study," *Biological Psychiatry* 62, no. 6 (September 15, 2007): 652–657, doi: 10.1016/j.biopsych.2006.11.021, https://pubmed.ncbi.nlm.nih.gov/17445781/.

19. S. Jacob et al., "Oral Administration of RAC-Alpha-Lipoic Acid Modulates Insulin Sensitivity in Patients with Type-2 Diabetes Mellitus: A Placebo-Controlled Pilot Trial," *Free Radical Biology & Medicine* 27, no. 3–4 (August 1999): 309–314, https://pubmed.ncbi.nlm.nih.gov/10468203/.

20. Amy M. Naleid et al., "Deconstructing the Vanilla Milkshake: The Dominant Effect of Sucrose on Self-Administration of Nutrient-Flavor Mixtures," *Appetite* 50, no. 1 (January 2008): 128–138, https://www.ncbi.nlm.nih.gov/pmc/articles/PMC2266682/.

21. Daniel G. Amen, *Use Your Brain to Change Your Age* (New York: Three Rivers Press, 2012), 146–150.

22. Jon Vezner and Randy Sharp, "Then What?" performed by Clay Walker on *Rumor Has It* album, Giant Records, © 1997.

## SECTION 7: THE DRAGON TAMER

1. Amen, *Change Your Brain, Change Your Life*, 5.

2. See my other books on brain health: *Change Your Brain, Change Your Life*, rev. ed. (New York: Harmony Books, 2015); *The Brain Warrior's Way* (New York: New American Library, 2016); and *The End of Mental Illness* (Carol Stream, IL: Tyndale, 2020).

3. Anders Wåhlin and Lars Nyberg, "At the Heart of Cognitive Functioning in Aging," *Trends in Cognitive Sciences* 23, no. 9 (September 2019): 717–720.

4. Cyrus A. Raji, et al. "Clinical Utility of SPECT Neuroimaging in the Diagnosis and Treatment of Traumatic Brain Injury: A Systematic Review," *PLOS ONE* 9, no. 3 (2014): e91088, https://www.ncbi.nlm.nih.gov/pmc/articles/PMC3960124/.

5. "Sleep and Sleep Disorder Statistics," American Sleep Association, 2020, https://sleepassociation.org/about-sleep/sleep-statistics/.

6. Hui Lei et al., "Altered Spontaneous Brain Activity in Obsessive-Compulsive Personality Disorder," *Comprehensive Psychiatry* 96, (January 2020): 152144.

7. Read more about the symptoms of ADD/ADHD in chapter 2 of *Healing ADD*, rev. ed. (New York: Berkley, 2013).

8. I first wrote about this exercise in *Change Your Brain, Change Your Life* (New York: Harmony Books, 2015).

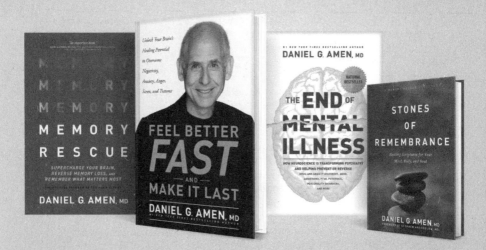